FUELLING THE
GAELIC ATHLETE

Fuelling the Gaelic Athlete: How to Optimise Your Nutrition to Improve Your Body Composition and Performance as an Athlete Involved in GAA Sports

First Published by Know Yourself Performance Ltd. 2021

Written by Conor O'Neill 2021

Text Copyright © Conor O'Neill 2021

Conor O'Neill has asserted his moral rights to be identified as the author of this work in accordance with the Copyright, Designs and Patents Act of 1988.

www.knowyourselfperformance.com

FUELLING THE GAELIC ATHLETE

How to Optimise Your Nutrition to Improve Your Body Composition
and Performance as an Athlete Involved in GAA Sports

By Conor O'Neill

CONTENTS

CONTENTS   4

ABOUT THE AUTHOR   8

PROLOGUE: 2 PARADOXES   10

Paradox 1: Improving Body Composition vs. Fuelling for Performance   10

Paradox 2: Perfect vs. Sustainable   13

INTRODUCTION: THE HIERARCHY OF NUTRITION   16

CHAPTER 1: THE NUMBERS GAME PART 1 – CALORIES   19

In Some Ways, Your Body is Like a Car   19

The Energy Balance Equation   21

But You're Not a Car   22

The Calculations   23

Example Calculation   25

What Rate of Progress Should You be Aiming for?   26

CHAPTER 2: THE NUMBERS GAME PART 2 - MACRONUTRIENTS   29

If it Fits Your Macros   30

Getting Accurate   31

Do I Need to Track all This?   32

Macro #1: Protein   33

Macro #2: Fat   34

Macro #3: Carbohydrates   36

Summary of Calculations   38

CHAPTER 3: THE NUMBERS GAME PART 3 - TRACKING YOUR FOOD INTAKE   41

Levels of Tracking   42

How to Track   43

Getting Accurate   44

CHAPTER 4: THE NUMBERS GAME PART 4 - ADJUSTING YOUR FOOD INTAKE   48

Adjusting Based on Progress   49

How Much to Adjust by?   51

Another Option: Adjusting Your Output   52

The Decision Tree   53

CHAPTER 5: MICRONUTRIENTS & FIBRE   55

Fruit and Vegetables   55

CHAPTER 6: MANAGING APPETITE   63

Decreasing Hunger   63

Getting More Food in   67

CHAPTER 7: HYDRATION   71

Fluid balance: Fluid out vs. Fluid in   71

Fluid Out   71

Fluid In   73

Negative Effects of Dehydration   73

1. Heart Rate   73

2. Temperature Regulation   74

3. Electrolyte Levels   74

The Rare Case of "Over-Hydration" (Hyponatremia)   75

Practical Implications   76

General Daily intake   76

During Training/Matches   77

After Training/Matches   77

CHAPTER 8: SLEEP   78

Performance   79

Fat-loss   79

Muscle Gain   79

Health   80

How Much Sleep Do You Need?   80

Tips For Better Sleep   81

CHAPTER 9: HOW MANY MEALS PER DAY?   84

Does it Actually Matter?   85

When it Does Matter   86

Appetite Management   86

Schedule   87

Muscle Protein Synthesis (MPS)   88

Eating Around Training and Matches   88

CHAPTER 10: EATING ON TRAINING VS. NON-TRAINING DAYS   90

Defining Your Days   91

Should You Use This Approach?   92

How Much Extra Should You Eat?   93

Adjusting Your Macronutrients   94

CHAPTER 11: CARBOHYDRATE LOADING   97

Carbohydrates for Sport   97

What is Carb-Loading?   98

Who Does it Work For?   99

How to Do it   100

Avoiding Common Mistakes and Problems   101

It's Not an Excuse to Eat Whatever You Want   101

Digestive Issues   102

CHAPTER 12: THE PRE-MATCH MEAL   104

It's Not Just About the Pre-match Meal   105

Game Day   106

The Pre-Match Meal   106

1. 1-4 Hours Pre-Match   107

2. 0-60 Minutes Pre-Match   109

CHAPTER 13: INTRA-PERFORMANCE NUTRITION   111

Fuelling   111

Hydration   113

Protein   114

The Ultimate Home-Made Intra-Performance Drink   115

Train Low?   116

CHAPTER 14: RECOVERY NUTRITION   118

Recovering   120

Rebuilding   120

Refuelling   121

Rehydrating   123

The Recovery "Window"   123

CHAPTER 15: MEAL PLANNING   125

A Word on Meal Plans   125

How to Plan Your Own Meals   127

Example Meal Plans   129

    1750 kcal   129

    2000 kcal   129

    2250 kcal   130

    2500 kcal   130

    2750 kcal   130

    3000 kcal   131

    3250 kcal   131

    3500 kcal   131

CHAPTER 16: SUPPLEMENTS   133

Protein Powder   134

Carbohydrate Supplements   135

Creatine   136

Caffeine   137

Fish Oil   139

Vitamin D   140

Magnesium & Zinc   140

Vitamin C   141

Multivitamin   142

Beta Alanine   143

Citrulline Malate   144

Beetroot Juice   145

Collagen Hydrolysate/Gelatin   145

CHAPTER 17: BRINGING IT ALL TOGETHER: THE ONE-PAGE NUTRITION PLAN   147

CONCLUDING REMARKS: IT'S OVER TO YOU   148

A Major Favour – And Something Extra for You   149

Where to go From Here   150

Bibliography   151

ABOUT THE AUTHOR

I was about 7 years old when my parents took me to my local GAA pitch in Crossmaglen for the first time. That was the start of a sporting journey through underage club teams, school teams, underage county academies, and eventually playing senior football, where I was honoured to play as part of a successful All-Ireland Club Championship winning team. My experience of playing (and perhaps my attempts to overcompensate for my mediocre skill level) led to me looking for methods of optimising my off-pitch approach, with nutrition and individual training being the obvious opportunities there. This led me down a path of obsession around how to optimise body composition and performance for athletic pursuits, particularly GAA. This obsession developed into a drive to become qualified to help others do the same.

To date, I've helped over 1000 athletes (most of whom are GAA players) with optimising their body composition and athletic performance, through improving their approach to nutrition and training. This book is a culmination of what I've learnt on the nutrition side of that equation. It comprises of a combination of what I've learnt from studying scientific literature, and practical experience gained from working with individuals and teams.

I hope that you find it useful in your pursuit of athletic success, and I hope that bleeds into improving every area of your life.

Conor O'Neill

PROLOGUE:

2 PARADOXES

Before beginning to discuss what foods you should be eating, what supplements you should be taking, how many litres of water you should be drinking, and all that good stuff, I want to introduce you to 2 paradoxes that any GAA player hoping to improve their nutrition will inevitably come up against. Recognising how to balance each of these paradoxes will likely change the way you approach your athletic goals, and will set the stage for the rest of the information in the book.

Paradox 1: Improving Body Composition vs. Fuelling for Performance

Body composition refers to the various types of bodily tissues that your body is composed of. From a general viewpoint these include muscle, body fat, bone, organs, and to some extent, even things like hair, nails, and skin. However, in the context of nutrition and training interventions, body composition generally relates to the amount of muscle mass a person has compared to the amount of body fat that person has, since these are the two that we often want to manipulate. Improving body composition, therefore, usually refers to some combination of reducing body fat and increasing muscle mass (outside of a few rare situations where body fat might be too low, or muscle mass might be too high for a given goal).

It is often presumed that efforts to improve body composition will be coupled with a decrease in athletic performance. This is backed up by many athletes who have tried severely decreasing their food intake whilst often increasing their training load (e.g., Implementing a low-carb diet whilst running extra laps of the field every night). You might have even tried a version of this yourself. These approaches can achieve the fat-loss goal in the short term, but at the expense of performance, since this person likely won't be providing enough fuel for their training demands. On the other side, efforts to improve body composition through increasing muscle mass can lead to overeating and subsequent body fat gain, which in turn can have negative consequences on performance. To illustrate this, imagine carrying around a 5kg weighted vest for every training session. Instead of that weighted vest, imagine you'd gained 5kg of body fat in a short time and had to carry that about the pitch.

Also, athletes hoping to optimally fuel for performance can have similar struggles affecting body composition. Athletes often struggle with their efforts to decrease body fat because they are trying to make sure they're eating enough to fuel each training session, for example. They also struggle to justify doing the gym sessions required for building muscle, since they worry about their ability to recover in time for training sessions and matches.

These struggles are completely understandable. Without a structured plan that considers both your body composition and performance-fuelling goals, based on the principles of scientific literature and practical application, you have no choice but to lean towards either extreme measures, or shooting in the dark. The problem is that when you're trying to balance these two goals, it's unproductive to go to extremes as outlined by the previous examples. Instead, you need to find the fine line where you're moving towards your body composition goals, whilst still fuelling for your performance demands. This requires a level of accuracy around what you're eating and what training you're doing, so that you're no longer shooting in the dark and hoping for the best.

With the hundreds of athletes I've worked with, from intercounty stars to the player hoping to get on the starting 15 of his division 3 club team, I've seen that when we get this balance right, the paradox flips on its head, where improving your body composition actually improves your performance, and vice versa, rather than both goals taking away from each other. By getting leaner and building more muscle, you improve your strength to weight ratio, potentially allowing for greater ability to sprint and jump. Perhaps you start going into tackles more confidently. Maybe you start taking on your opponent more often. The confidence that comes with improved body composition can have psychological benefits too. Improving your fuelling can also allow you to recover more quickly and train more often (allowing for those extra gym sessions to build muscle) and can also decrease the worry that athletes often have of 'wasting muscle' because of the high cardiovascular training load, thereby further improving body composition. I've seen the effects of getting this balance right first-hand with the athletes I've worked with, and this book is written to get that information out to as many people who need it as possible.

Paradox 2: Perfect vs. Sustainable

The second paradox involves the balance between what would be a perfect approach in a perfect world and what is a sustainable approach that actually makes sense for you and your lifestyle. In other words, "What you should do if the circumstances were perfect" vs. "What you will actually do consistently given your current circumstances". As an example, you could be given the perfect meal plan for your goals from a body composition and performance point of view, but if the foods on that plan are out of your budget, are foods that you don't enjoy, and require you to eat at times that don't suit your schedule, it's only a matter of time before you give it up altogether and go back to your former eating habits, those that weren't moving you towards your goals. Contrast that with an approach that is 90% optimal for your goals, but allows you a bit more flexibility with meal timing, includes foods that you enjoy and eat regularly, allows you to fit in social occasions, and suits your budget constraints. You're much more likely to keep that way of eating up for much longer than the 'perfect' approach, which is far more likely to lead to better results over the long-term. A 'good' diet for 6 months is going to lead to far greater progress than a 'perfect' diet for 2 weeks.

The balance between these two can be seen as a sliding scale. A lot of where you start on this scale will be based on what your current approach is. For example, if you're someone who currently eats fast food 3-4 times per week, only eats a couple of portions of vegetables each week, and has no idea of what a protein source is, simply aiming to include 3 portions of veg each day, reduce fast food intake to once per week, and have 2-3 protein sources per day is likely to be enough to lead to progress, without being so far away from your current approach to cause it to be unsustainable. Over time, someone in this position can progress to a more advanced approach, but to go straight to food tracking, carb-loading, advanced supplementation, and similarly advanced approaches is likely to be too overwhelming straight off the bat, leading to unsustainability and inevitable failure. But if you're someone who already tracks your food intake regularly, eats protein and vegetables with each meal, drinks adequate fluids, and utilises the basic supplements for your goals already, looking at more specific and minute details could well be sustainable for you, and could lead to getting that extra few percentage points of progress out of your approach, even though doing so might seem ridiculously complicated and unsustainable to someone else.

For these reasons, taking this paradox into account when considering any changes to your current approach is likely to lead to more progress over time. To give a specific example: when considering whether to have differing intakes on training vs. non-training days, it's important to consider the fact that this is adding an element of complication. Adding that element might be worth it to you if you know you can maintain it over time, but if you're currently unable to hit the same intake consistently each day, adding that element is likely to make your approach even more difficult, leading to you giving it up completely. The same is true for carb-loading, adding supplements, increasing fruit and vegetable intake, and any other changes you might consider.

As a summary to this section, remember that consistency is more important than perfection. Get started, even with an approach that is sustainable for you, even if it isn't completely perfect, and aim to make small improvements to that approach over time. With those things in mind, you're ready to start getting stuck in.

INTRODUCTION:

THE HIERARCHY OF

NUTRITION

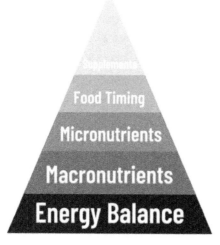

If you've previously tried to improve your nutrition, you'll probably

have noticed the minefield of information that is out there in books, in conversation, and on the internet. This can leave you at a complete loss as to where to start and what to do. Fortunately, there are many people out there who have worked to simplify this and construct approaches and systems to help.

One example of this is the Eric Helms' Nutrition Pyramid, which breaks down the key components of a good nutrition plan, in hierarchical order. This means that the elements are arranged so that the most important element is at the bottom, and the least important element is at the top, with those elements in between arranged accordingly.

This can give you an idea of where to start with nutritional changes to get the most out of your efforts, but can also allow you to assess how important a given nutrition intervention might be, given your current level of nutrition. For example, if you are considering implementing a strategy of changing your meal timing (e.g. optimising your pre-training meal), you could look at the pyramid and notice that food timing is quite close to the top of the pyramid. This means that if you haven't already implemented changes in the levels below that (Energy balance, macronutrients, and micronutrients), then you might be better suited addressing those issues first.

This book is somewhat based around this pyramid, and you'll notice the order of chapters are set out in a similar order to what you'd expect from looking at the pyramid. There are a couple of chapters in this book that aren't specifically outlined on the pyramid (e.g., sleep and hydration), but these will be slotted in in order of importance for the most part.

The 'Energy balance' portion of the pyramid will cover the amount of energy (measured in calories) that one consumes vs. the amount of energy expended through everyday life and training, and the implications that can have on body composition and performance. The 'Macronutrients' portion will cover the breakdown of your energy intake into the components protein, fat, and carbohydrates. 'Micronutrients' will cover fruit and vegetable intake, but appetite management, hydration, and sleep also align with this theme. 'Food timing' will comprise of aspects like carb-loading, altering your daily intake based on training load, and eating around training and matches. The 'Supplements' section will then outline some supplements for you to consider and how you might go about implementing these.

With all this said, the book is designed to be read in the order in which the chapters are laid out, but can also be used as a reference tool if and when you have a specific aspect of nutrition that you're choosing to focus on. The action points at the end of each chapter should be completed in order to get the most out of each chapter. The 'One-page Nutrition Plan' at the end of the book then aims to bring all the action points into one reference point that you can use to outline your complete nutritional approach and to keep you focussed on what to do over time.

CHAPTER 1:

THE NUMBERS GAME

PART 1 – CALORIES

"I eat well, but still can't get rid of this extra body fat."

"I eat a lot, but just can't gain weight."

"I'm not sure if I'm eating enough to fuel my sports performance and gym-work."

These sentiments are frequently expressed by athletes who are struggling to adapt their nutrition to suit their body composition and performance goals. Generally, the issue here is one of specificity.

In Some Ways, Your Body is Like a Car

To over-simplify it, the body is, in some ways, like a car, in that it requires a certain amount of fuel and a certain type of fuel in order for it to optimally do the job you're asking it to. For example, if you were asking someone to put fuel in your car, you wouldn't just tell them to "Put a lot of fuel in", or "Use good fuel", you would tell them how much to put in, based on how much travelling you were planning on doing, and you'd tell them the exact type of fuel needed (diesel or petrol, for example) based on which type of fuel was right for your specific car. Similarly, leaving the fuelling of your body open to vague terms like "A lot" or "Well" can lead to sub-par results.

Of course, the quality of food that you fuel your body with is important (we'll get to that in upcoming chapters), but in the same way that even high-quality diesel won't get you to where you want to go if you don't have enough of it, the best quality of food won't be enough to fuel you if you don't eat the right amount of it. For car fuel, the numbers we use are usually litres or the monetary equivalent. The food we eat contains energy, and that energy is measured in calories, so the number of calories contained in foods is the main number we use when talking about fuelling the body - that's the equivalent of the number of litres of fuel. This can refer to the energy we put into our body through food, and the energy we use through exercise and daily life. These two aspects form what's known as the energy balance equation.

The Energy Balance Equation

The energy intake side of the equation is made up of the food and drink that you consume. The energy output side of things can be broken down into various elements (It isn't crucial that you know these, so if it feels overcomplicated, simply skip this paragraph). The main contributor to the energy output side of the equation is your resting metabolic rate (RMR), which is the energy used to keep the body alive at rest. On top of that, there is the thermic effect of feeding (TEF) which is the energy used to digest the food you eat, non-exercise activity thermogenesis (NEAT) which is the energy used in everyday activities outside of exercise (walking about, tying your shoelaces, brushing your teeth etc,) and exercise activity thermogenesis (EAT), which is the energy used during exercise. Again, unless you're an enthusiast of nutrition, all you need to take away from this is that the food you take in provides your energy intake, and your energy output is comprised of what is needed to keep your body alive, digest your food, fuel your daily activity, and fuel your exercise/training.

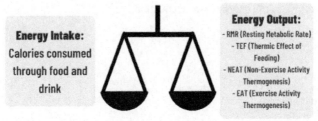

Energy Intake:
Calories consumed through food and drink

Energy Output:
- RMR (Resting Metabolic Rate)
- TEF (Thermic Effect of Feeding)
- NEAT (Non-Exercise Activity Thermogenesis)
- EAT (Exercise Activity Thermogenesis)

If the amount of energy you take in (through food and drinks) is greater than the amount you use/burn on average (the sum of each of the aforementioned aspects), you will be in a state of **energy surplus, or calorie surplus**, the extra energy will be stored, and you will gain weight over time.

If the amount of energy you use/burn is greater than the amount you take in on average, you will be in a state of **energy deficit, or calorie deficit**, your body will use its energy stores (from body fat, for example) to get the energy it needs, and you will lose weight over time.

If the amount of energy you take in is the same as the amount you use/burn on average, you will be in a state of **maintenance**, where you are supplying enough energy to fuel your body (no more, no less) and you will remain the same weight over time.

Simply put, the amount of energy that you take in vs. the amount you output will determine whether you lose, gain, or maintain body weight.

But You're Not a Car

Although we can draw some conclusions about the body based on its similarity to a car, it isn't a car, and doesn't work in exactly the same way. One way in which this is true is that, for the body, one side of the energy equation can have a significant effect on the other. This topic could make up a chapter in itself and would contain more detail than would be practical, but I'll give a couple of quick examples. If you were to eat in a calorie deficit for a period of time, and therefore lose weight, you will now have less body mass to carry around. Your body will need to use less energy on a daily basis to carry this now-lighter body, meaning that you will probably need to eat slightly less to lose the same amount of weight from there on in. On the other end of the scale, if you eat in a surplus over time, and gain weight, you now have more body weight to carry around. Your energy output increases, potentially creating a situation where you need to eat more in order to gain the same amount of weight going forward. You also may unconsciously start to move more, train harder etc, as your body "finds stuff to do" with all this extra energy (although storing fat may still be one of those things). The same is true for someone who is eating less in order to lose weight, where they may unconsciously start to move less (with some studies even showing that people start blinking less when in an energy deficit), decreasing their energy output in the process. It's important to note that some people are more sensitive than others to these effects.

Based on that, plus the fact that training load and activity levels change throughout the weeks and months, it would be impossible to calculate an exact figure for how much energy you will be expending, and therefore how much you should be eating. So, instead of thinking we can calculate the exact amount, we use the best estimates we can, and adjust over time.

The Calculations

In order to calculate your TDEE (total daily energy expenditure), and furthermore, your recommended calorie intake, there are many equations used in the scientific literature and in practice, and they can all get quite complicated. Here's one that's basic enough to calculate for yourself, whilst giving you a good estimate to start with.

Step 1: Multiply your bodyweight in kg by 22-24:

> BW (in kg) x 22 for those with relatively low activity outside of training.
>
> BW (in kg) x 23 for those with moderate activity outside of training.
>
> BW (in kg) x 24 for those with relatively high activity outside of training.

Step 2: Multiply the answer from step 1 by an activity multiplier, based on your training load:

> If you are sedentary (little or no exercise): 'Answer from step 1' x 1.2
>
> If you are lightly active (Train 1-3 days/week): 'Answer from step 1' x 1.35
>
> If you are moderately active (Train 3-5 days/week): 'Answer from step 1' x 1.55
>
> If you are very active (Train hard 6-7 days a week): 'Answer from step 1' x 1.7
>
> If you are extremely active (Train very hard every day & physical job or train 2x/day) : 'Answer from step 1' x 1.9

Step 3: Decrease or increase based on bodyweight loss/gain goal:
For weight-loss:

Decrease by 10-20% (towards the lower end if performance is a priority, towards the higher end if weight-loss is a priority)

For weight-gain:

Increase by 5-10% (towards the lower end if staying lean is a priority, towards the higher end if weight-gain is a priority)

You could increase the deficit/surplus beyond these recommendations in certain situations, but these are good starting points.

Example Calculation

Let's take, for example, an 80kg footballer, who trains 3 times per week, with two gym sessions, is relatively active (has an office job, but does a decent amount of walking around the office and has a 15-minute walk to and from work) and wants to gain weight.

Step 1: Bodyweight in kg x 23

80 x 23 (based on his/her moderate activity level)

= 1840 kcal

Step 2: 'Answer from step 1' x Activity Multiplier

1840 x 1.55 (based on him/her training 3-5 times per week)

= 2852 kcal (this would be his/her estimated maintenance)

Step 3: 'Answer from step 2' + Percentage based on weight goals

2852 + 10% of 2852 (based on weight gain goal)

2852 + 285

= 3137

= 3150 kcal (rounded)

What Rate of Progress Should You be Aiming for?

Before getting into bodyweight progress targets, it's important to note that bodyweight isn't by any means the only measure of progress. We'll cover this more as we go through the progress tracking chapter, but you can imagine a case where you're trying to get leaner, and bodyweight isn't moving much, but you're looking leaner, feeling lighter on your feet and performing better. If you were to look only at body weight in this situation, you might think progress is going slowly, when in fact, you're making huge strides. Even so, bodyweight can be a useful metric to keep track of, since it can inform you of your energy balance status (whether you are in an energy deficit or surplus, or at maintenance level, on average), thus helping inform your decisions, along with the other progress metrics you're aiming to improve. With that said, here are some general guidelines that are worth considering:

- Fat-loss: Aim to reduce body weight by 0.5-1% per week. (e.g., Losing 0.4-0.8kg per week for an 80kg athlete. Towards the lower end if performance is a priority, towards the higher end if weight-loss is a priority).

- Maintenance: Aim to remain the same bodyweight as time goes on. This can be useful if someone is hoping to gain muscle and drop body fat during the same period. This is known as body re-composition, and is more applicable to someone who is new to weight-training, or has been away from it from a long time. Intermediate or advanced trainees would be better suited to focussing on fat-loss or muscle gain specifically for a period of time.
- Muscle Gain: Aim to increase bodyweight by 1-2% per month. (e.g., Gaining 0.8-1.6kg per month for an 80kg athlete. Towards the lower end if staying lean is a priority, towards the higher end if weight-gain is a priority).

Over time, through tracking your progress, you'll begin to see if you are making progress in this fashion. If not, you'll have to adjust over time, as shown in chapter 4. Before that though, we need to look at what your daily calories will be made up of, by looking at the macronutrient breakdown.

Calculating Your Calorie Targets

Here are the steps for you to take to calculate your calorie targets. Use the information in the chapter to inform where you fall within each range:

1. Multiply your bodyweight by 22-24 based on your everyday activity: _____kcal

2. Multiply your answer from step 1 by 1.2-1.9 based on your training level: _____kcal

3. Add or subtract 5-20% to/from your answer from step 2 based on your weight loss/gain goal: _____kcal

Your daily calorie intake target (answer from step 3): _____kcal

CHAPTER 2:

THE NUMBERS

GAME PART 2 -

MACRONUTRIENTS

Simply focussing on hitting your calorie intake targets will allow you to move your bodyweight in the right direction, and for someone who is interested in simply losing weight or gaining weight, that might be enough. But for athletes, who generally want to ensure that any body weight reduction is in the form of body fat, or any weight gain to be in the form or muscle, and who want to make sure they're optimally fuelling their body for their performance demands, getting a bit more specific with where those calories come from is going to be important. And that's where looking at the macronutrient breakdown (protein, fat, and carbohydrates) of those calories comes into play.

If it Fits Your Macros

The concept of individuals tracking their macronutrient intake in order to optimise body composition and performance seems to have been popularised by bodybuilders in the early 2000s. The approach before that was to simply focus on eating 'clean' foods, with the common trope of unseasoned boiled chicken, rice, and broccoli often being held up as a typical good bodybuilding meal. As sports science progressed and made its way into the sport of bodybuilding, some began to realise that as long as they were hitting certain daily macronutrient (protein, fat, and carbohydrate) goals, they could be flexible in their food choices, without the need to stick to the boring foods of previous generations. For example, leaving out some of the rice from their dinner allowed them to enjoy a bowl of cereal after dinner, allowing them to hit the same carbohydrate target, whilst including a food they enjoyed. This approach became known as an 'If it fits your macros" (IIFYM) approach. Subsequently, some would say that the pendulum started to swing the other way, where many bodybuilders (and subsequently many everyday trainees) began to see this as freedom to eat in a way that disregarded quality of food almost completely, knowing that as long as their foods 'fit their macros', regardless of whether that was from fresh whole foods or confectionery and take-aways, they'd progress with their body composition goals. Whilst this may be true, it's certainly not an optimal approach, for many other reasons, to disregard the quality of food you're eating (more on that in future chapters). However, you can take lessons from this, namely that you can include some of the foods you enjoy, even if they're not typically seen as 'clean' or optimally healthy foods, and doing so in a way that fits into your calorie and macronutrient goals for the day will allow for much greater progress than if you hadn't adjusted around these meals. This element of flexibility will also allow for greater adherence to your nutritional plan over the long-term, since you won't feel as if you're completely restricting yourself to a specific set of foods.

Getting Accurate

The flexibility side of tracking your macronutrient intake is one thing, but what we're really seeking with this approach is a level of accuracy that would otherwise be very difficult to achieve. Sports science has given us solid data around what amounts of foods we should be consuming on a daily basis in order to optimise for our goals, so if you want to use that to its fullest, an element of tracking your food intake (at least for a period of time) is going to be useful.

The three main macronutrients - protein, fat, and carbohydrates - make up your daily energy intake, meaning that by manipulating your macronutrient intake, you are also manipulating your energy intake/calorie intake. (Alcohol is technically a fourth macronutrient, but we'll not discuss it as much here, since it makes up such a small fraction of most people's daily intake.)

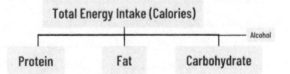

Do I Need to Track all This?

Of course, you don't *need* to track your macronutrients, but if you're really wanting to optimise your body composition and performance, it definitely helps. Otherwise, you're not going to know if you're actually hitting the recommended targets. For most athletes, tracking for at least a period of a few weeks/months will be a useful exercise. If nothing else, this will give you an insight into what macronutrients are contained within the foods you are eating currently, as well as giving you an insight into how different your current intake might be to a more optimal one. From there, you can choose to continue tracking and maintaining that level of accuracy, or you can simply make habit based changes to get you closer to a more suitable macronutrient intake (e.g. if you realise you're consistently hitting less than your protein target, you may simply decide to add an extra portion of a protein-rich food to each meal). Also, whether you regularly track your food or not can depend, in part, on how it fits into your lifestyle and your relationship with food. Some people find it quite constricting and impractical, whereas others find it frees them up, knowing that they can fit in some treats, whilst fuelling their training and achieving their body composition goals. Either way, having a good knowledge of what each macronutrient does, and having a good idea of how much you, as an individual, should be consuming daily, is likely to lead to improved performance and body composition.

Macro #1: Protein

When you eat protein-rich foods, the protein is broken down into smaller particles, known as amino acids. These amino acids are the building blocks of protein structures such as muscle tissue, as well as other bodily tissues like hair and nails. Our muscles are constantly in a state of flux, meaning that they are being broken down (and not just through exercise) and built back up simultaneously. In order to ensure the building up (synthesis) of new muscle equals or exceeds the breakdown, it is important to supply the body with sufficient amino acids, by eating enough protein through food. Doing regular resistance training (e.g. lifting weights) will also increase the muscle synthesis (building) side of this equation.

Generally, the amount of protein you require will rely on how much training you are doing, and how much muscle mass you have (which roughly correlates with your body weight.) For most athletes, a recommendation of 2g of protein per kg of body weight is a good target, based on studies investigating what is optimal for muscle synthesis and recovery. For example, for an athlete weighing 80kg, this will be:

80 x 2 = 160g of protein per day

To put that in context, here are a few common protein sources with how many grams of protein they contain (based on average sizes of each source):

- Medium chicken breast: 30-40g

- 4 eggs: 24g
- 1 Scoop whey protein: 20-25g
- Medium steak: 60-80g
- Salmon fillet: 30-40g
- Pot of Greek yoghurt: 19g

In order to see how that fits into the overall calorie intake equation, let's say this 80kg athlete had an estimated calorie requirement of 3000 kcal. Given that protein contains 4 kcal per gram, we can say that this athlete is getting 640 kcal (that's 160 x 4) out of their 3000 kcal daily total from protein.

That leaves 2360 kcal (3000 - 640) to be split between fat and carbohydrates.

(Note: If all this maths seems confusing to you, don't worry, there will be a section at the end of the chapter that guides you through how to calculate your own, as well as a table where you don't even have to calculate them. Skip the maths here if you want.)

Macro #2: Fat

When we eat foods containing dietary fat, the fat is broken down into fatty acids, which can be used for energy, or stored for energy in adipose tissue (body fat) for later use. That doesn't mean you have to do star-jumps every time you eat some fat in order to avoid fat gain, however. As with our muscle protein, our body fat is continuously in flux, with fatty acids continuously being both released to be burned as energy, and being stored. The balance of how much is released and burned vs. how much is stored is ultimately what determines how much body fat is gained overall. This is almost completely a result of how much energy (calories) you take in vs. how much you expend/burn (energy balance) over time. Fat is also used in the regulation of hormones and the maintenance of cell structures, as well as the absorption of fat-soluble vitamins A,D,E, and K. In calculating how much fat you should be aiming to consume, it's important to consume enough to cover the body's requirements to carry out these processes and the other biological processes involving fat. Fat also contributes to the overall enjoyability of the diet, which is important when considering the sustainability of the diet. On the other hand, it's also important to remember that the more fat you consume, the fewer carbohydrates you'll be able to consume whilst staying within your calorie target, and given the importance of carbohydrates for athletic performance, you may not want to have to overly reduce your intake of them.

With all these things considered, starting somewhere in the range of 0.8-1.2g per kg body weight is likely close to optimal based on the scientific literature. You could go towards the higher or lower end of that range based on preference. For those aiming for a relatively low-calorie intake target (in a fat-loss phase for example), it would likely be better to edge towards the lower end, in order to allow room for enough carbohydrates and protein to be consumed, whilst staying within your caloric target. For those aiming for a relatively high calorie intake target (in a muscle gain phase for example), it would likely be better to edge towards the higher end of the fat intake range in order to make it easier to hit the calorie target, since fat sources are higher in calories than protein or carbohydrates.

For our 80kg athlete, that is 64-96g of fat daily (80 x 0.8-1.2), so 80g would be a good place to start.

To put that in context, here are some examples of how much fat is in various foods:

- 30g cashew nuts: 12g
- 30g dark chocolate:10g
- 1 egg: 5g
- 1 fillet of salmon: 20g
- 1 tablespoon olive oil: 14g

Given that fat contains 9kcal per gram, we can say that fat will contribute 720 kcal (80 x 9) to our example athlete's overall diet.

This means that protein and fat will contribute 1360 kcal total (640+720) out of the 3000 kcal this 80kg athlete needs, leaving 1640 kcal (3000-1360) for carbohydrates.

(Again, don't worry if the maths goes over your head.)

Macro #3: Carbohydrates

When you eat carbohydrate-rich foods, the carbohydrates are broken down into glucose (sugar). This is true whether this carbohydrate comes from sweet potatoes or a donut. This glucose is then circulated around the body, where it is either used to produce energy, or stored as glycogen (a name given to the stored form of carbohydrates), for when it's needed, in high-intensity training, for example. In rare cases, where an extreme amount of carbohydrates are ingested, the glucose can be converted and stored as fat, but this is usually only the case when this extremely high intake forces someone well over their calorie intake target. Given the high glycolytic (glucose-dependent) demands of GAA sports, where there is a lot of intermittent high-intensity running, for example, it is important to have high levels of glycogen stores in the muscles to optimise performance. This is achieved by consuming adequate levels of carbohydrates through food. There can also be benefits to increasing levels of blood glucose immediately before and during training and matches, which is achieved through adequate timing and quantities of carbohydrate intake (more on that in later chapters).

In terms of calculating your recommended intake, you have done most of the work by calculating how many calories are left after calculating your protein and fat targets. For the 80kg GAA athlete we've been using in this chapter, we calculated that there is 1640 kcal left for carbohydrates. Given that carbohydrates provide around 4 kcal per gram, this 1640 kcal is equal to about 410g (1640 / 4) of carbohydrate.

However, based on scientific research, we also know that somewhere in the region of 3.5-6.5 g of carbohydrate per day is likely to be optimal for mixed sports. We can use this figure as a check on the previous calculation. For our 80kg athlete, this range is 280-520g.

In this case, our target falls within this range, so we will stick with it. However, there may be cases where our calculations give us recommendations outside of this range, so we may need to manipulate other factors to get closer to this range. For example, you may choose to decrease our fat intake target to allow us more carbohydrates whilst staying within our calorie target.

For context, here are some examples of carbohydrate sources with the amount of carbohydrates in each:

- 100g rice (raw weight): 75g
- 400g potatoes: 68g
- 100g pasta (raw weight): 75g
- 2 slices of bread: 32g
- 1 sports drink: 32g
- 3 rice cakes: 20g
- 1 large sweet potato: 30-40g

Summary of Calculations

For our 80kg athlete (for whom we calculated a target of 3000kcal/day):

- Protein: 2g per kg bodyweight = 2 x 80 = **160g/day**
- Fat: 0.8-1.2g per kg bodyweight = 0.8-1.2 x 80 = 64-96g/day = **80g/day** as a middle ground
- Carbohydrate: The rest of the calories = 1640 kcal / 4 = **410g/day** (should also be in the range of 3.5-6.5 g per kg bodyweight = 3.5-6.5 x 80 = 280-520g/day).

Alternatively, if that maths all seems a bit much to you, you can check out the chart below to give you a rough estimate of your starting point based on your bodyweight.

Body Weight (St & lb) >		8 st 9 lb	9 st 6 lb	10 st 3 lb	11st	11 st 11 lb	12 st 8 lb	13 st 5 lb	14 st 2 lb	14 st 13 lb	15 st 10 lb
Body Weight (kg) >		55	60	65	70	75	80	85	90	95	100
Weight-Loss	Calories	1850	1950	2050	2150	2250	2300	2350	2450	2550	2650
	Protein	130	135	140	150	160	165	175	185	200	210
	Fat	55	60	60	60	65	65	65	70	75	75
	Carbohydrates	210	220	240	260	260	265	265	265	270	285
Weight Maintenance	Calories	2160	2250	2350	2450	2550	2640	2730	2820	2900	3000
	Protein	120	125	135	145	155	160	170	190	200	210
	Fat	55	60	65	65	70	75	75	80	80	85
	Carbohydrates	300	300	310	320	330	335	340	340	350	350
Weight-Gain	Calories	2350	2500	2650	2750	2850	3000	3100	3250	3400	3500
	Protein	120	125	135	145	150	160	170	180	190	200
	Fat	60	65	70	75	80	85	85	90	95	100
	Carbohydrates	330	360	375	375	385	400	415	425	445	455

Note: These recommendations are based on estimates for someone who is aged between 20-30, 10-20% bodyfat, training 3-5 times per week, and moderately active in everyday life, so you may need to adjust based on your unique circumstances. (e.g. if you're very inactive and/or training less frequently, calorie recommendations should be decreased, and vice versa).

Action Point

Calculating Your Macronutrient Intake

Here are the steps for you to take to calculate your macronutrient targets:

1. Calculate your calorie intake target (from previous chapter): _____kcal

2. Multiply your current bodyweight (in kg) by 2 to get your protein target (in grams): _____g

3. Multiply your answer from step 2 by 4 in order to get the number of calories consumed by protein: _____ kcal

4. Multiply your current bodyweight (in kg) by 0.8-1.2 (1 for example) to get your fat target (in grams): _____g

5. Multiply that number by 9 in order to get the number of calories consumed by fat: _____ kcal

6. Look at your answer to number 1 (_____) and take away answer number 3 (_____) and number 5 (_____) to get the total calories left for carbohydrates: _____ kcal

7. Divide answer 6 by 4 in order to get your carbohydrate target in grams: _____g

Your targets:

Protein (answer from number 2): _____g

Fat (answer from number 5): _____g

Carbohydrates (answer from number 7): _____g

CHAPTER 3:

THE NUMBERS GAME

PART 3 - TRACKING

YOUR FOOD INTAKE

The obvious question that might come up at this stage is around how, knowing all these numbers, you might go about hitting them. There are a number of ways of doing so, with varying levels of accuracy and ease of use. In order to achieve a level of accuracy that is likely to lead to the improvements most people are hoping to see, most people will require some level of food tracking, at least for a period of time. This generally involves either writing down the food you eat each day or inputting it into an app, in order to assess your nutritional intake on a daily basis, allowing you to adjust it as needed. There are a multitude of different components of food that you could be looking at, to the point where it has the potential to become confusing. In this case, we want to balance what is optimal vs. what is sustainable for the period of time that you're going to be doing it. With that said, there is a range of options when it comes to what figures you should be paying attention to when tracking your food.

Levels of Tracking

On one end of the food tracking scale, you could opt to simply pay attention to the number of calories you are taking in, disregarding the macronutrients (protein, fat, and carbohydrate) for now. This approach will likely be better than not tracking at all, but will potentially lead to missing out on the previously mentioned benefits of hitting your macronutrient targets. That trade-off might be worth it for you if you're new to the food tracking process and want to get the process started without overcomplicating it. However, you may want to push things in the direction of optimality by then starting to include a focus on protein along with the calorie target. This will allow you to move bodyweight in the desired direction and likely cover your recovery and muscle building needs, but may see you missing out on some of the potential fuelling benefits of getting your carbohydrates and fats at an appropriate level. Finally, adding in that element of tracking carbohydrates and fats brings another level of accuracy, allowing you to reap those benefits.

As mentioned previously, how you choose to track, and what figures you choose to pay attention to, depends on a few aspects including what level of nutrition you're currently at and how much effort you're willing to put into ensuring your progress. For a beginner, a good approach is to bring these elements in in a progressive fashion, starting with focussing on hitting your calorie target for the first few weeks, then starting to also pay attention to your protein intake for the next few weeks, followed by starting to pay attention to carbohydrate and fat intake once you've been consistently hitting your calorie and protein targets for a few weeks. This means you will be progressing along the way with your body composition and performance, but will also be progressing with your nutritional approach as a whole.

So, the progression of levels of food tracking look like: Calories only → Calories and protein → Calories, protein, fats, and carbs.

How to Track

Regardless of what metrics you chose to keep an eye on, you're going to need to track the food that you are eating. This could be done by writing down the foods you are eating, searching the internet for the calorie and macronutrient contents of them, and adding them up to find your daily total, but technological advances mean that there are now much easier ways of tracking your daily intake and assessing how close you are to your daily targets. Phone apps like 'MyFitnessPal' and 'Chronometer' are excellent tools in this regard. These apps have databases of foods which allow you to search for specific foods within the app and enter the amount of that food that you've eaten. The app will automatically add that to your total intake for the day, as well as giving you an indication of how many calories and grams of each macronutrient you have left before hitting your daily targets. Each of the dozens of food tracking apps out there will have their pros and cons, so it's a good idea to play around with them and see which one best suits your needs and preferences.

Getting Accurate

The level of accuracy with which you will be able to hit your goals will also be based on how accurate you are with the data that you enter into the app. This firstly includes how diligent you are in ensuring that you are tracking every piece of food or drink that you consume. It can be quite common to underreport food intake consciously or unconsciously, to the extent that even registered dieticians mistakenly underreport their intake in clinical studies! This underreporting can be a result of simply forgetting to input full meals, but can also include leaving out small snacks, bites, spoonfuls, and drinks of things that you may think are too insignificant to track. Ultimately however, these things can add up to substantial differences over the course of a day or week, so it's important that for optimal accuracy, you track everything you eat and drink.

Another cause for inaccuracy is lack of accuracy in the amounts of the foods that you are tracking. If you are not weighing the individual ingredients, you can easily be off in terms of how much you're actually eating. For example, if you're tracking '1 chicken fillet', there is likely to be a level of inaccuracy, since chicken fillets vary in size and weight, and therefore calorie and macronutrient content. Instead, it would be much more accurate to weigh your chicken fillet and enter the amount in grams, giving a true reflection of the calorie and macronutrient content of that food.

Another common issue involves weighing food cooked vs. uncooked and tracking it as the other. Because water is generally added to some foods (think pasta or rice) and taken away from other foods (think vegetables or meat) during the cooking process, it is important to be consistent in tracking the food in the state you actually weighed it. For example, if you cook a 150g chicken fillet, it might lose 25g of water during the cooking process, and therefore weigh 125g when cooked. In this case, you're left with the dilemma of whether to use the 150g figure or the 125g figure. It is generally recommended that you weigh and track the food in the raw form, since this isn't subject to the length of cooking time, in the way that using the cooked weight would be, allowing for more consistency. But that isn't always possible, since sometimes you'll be buying your food already cooked. For that reason, the main recommendation here is that if you weigh it in the raw form, you track it in the raw form, and if you weigh it in the cooked form, you track it in the cooked form. This can usually be done quite simply by adding in the word 'raw' or 'cooked' when searching for the food in your food tracking app. E.g. Search: "Chicken raw", and then enter the weight of the chicken fillet when it was raw.

You may run into some difficulties when you're not the person cooking your food, or when you're cooking a large portion of food (for a family meal for example). In these cases, it will be about doing your best to give a good estimate of the food you're eating. It

45

won't be perfect, but will likely be better than if you hadn't tracked at all. Additionally, your ability to accurately estimate your intakes in these cases will be dependent on your previous tracking experience. You'll be much better at visually estimating what weight of rice you're eating, for example, if you've weighed and tracked rice dozens of times previously.

Your ability to accurately track your food will improve over time, and more than that, your ability to accurately hit your calorie and macronutrient targets will improve. The first few weeks of the tracking process will involve getting used to the app, as well as starting to observe how close or far away you are from the targets set out. As the weeks go on, you'll then begin to recognise where you are specifically over or under your targets, and by starting to look at what foods contribute to each of the metrics, you can start increasing or decreasing specific foods within your diet to adjust your intake, allowing you to get closer and closer to the targets over time.

Not only that, but you'll also start to develop a better instinct for what meals are conducive to your goals, and what a day of eating looks like when it comes to hitting your targets. Down the line, this will mean that you are able to be pretty close to your targets without needing to track everything to a tee, allowing you to move away from the tracking process as you see fit, and then take up tracking again as and when it is needed to dial your intake in for specific periods of time for specific targets.

Action Point

Getting Used to Tracking

Download 1-2 food tracking apps, and start navigating them, getting used to the process, and assessing which one might suit best for your food tracking going forward.

CHAPTER 4:

THE NUMBERS GAME

PART 4 - ADJUSTING

YOUR FOOD INTAKE

So we've gone through various stages to calculate estimates of the calorie and macronutrient intake targets required to get you moving in the direction of your goals. We've also gone through how to track your intake of food in order to hit those targets. It's important to reiterate, however, that these targets are estimates, based on the average requirements for someone of your physical attributes and goals. Therefore, it may be the case that these figures need to be adjusted to better suit your goals. In this case, these adjustments will be made based on your weekly progress. Whilst bodyweight isn't the only metric we care about, it is a really useful metric, particularly in a fat-loss or muscle gain context, since it is accessible (most people have a weighing scale in their house, but not many have a DEXA body fat scanner, for example), and it is a good proxy for body fat and muscle changes over time. It isn't the only thing you should track, as outlined below, and if you're someone who gets obsessive about scale weight when monitoring it, it may be worth leaving out and focussing on the other metrics discussed.

Adjusting Based on Progress

When you compare your actual weekly bodyweight progress to what you'd expected in your calculations, you can get an idea of whether or notyou need to adjust calories. E.g., If you're aiming to lose 0.5 kg per week, but after 3 weeks, you've only lost 0.3kg per week on average, it might be worth considering adjusting your calorie intake downwards to get to that 0.5kg per week average. There is a bit of nuance required here, however, in that whilst body weight is a great proxy measure for progress in a fat-loss phase, it doesn't tell the full story. E.g., If you set out to lose 0.5kg on average per week but are only losing 0.3kg on average per week, but you are seeing a lot of progress visually, and are feeling great in training, and are happy with your rate of progress, decreasing calorie intake might not be required at all. In fact, if that's the case, it may be better to stick with your current approach, allowing you to keep eating that higher calorie intake whilst being really happy with the progress you're making. It's also worth noting that the difference in these measurements can easily be down to rounding errors and fluctuations, so it's worth measuring your weight multiple times per week, at the same time and in the same conditions, and then taking a weekly average, using that as your progress metric.

The need to change your calorie and macronutrient target is more applicable in cases where your actual progress is very different to your goal. E.g. If you are aiming to lose 0.5kg per week, and weight hasn't moved at all in 3-4 weeks, or worse yet, you've gained weight, that is a good sign that you'll probably benefit from decreasing your intake targets. This concept also applies to those aiming to gain weight. If you're aiming to gain 0.3kg per week, and the scales haven't moved in 3-4 weeks, it's probably time to move your calorie intake up. Again, visual changes can be indicative that calorie changes may not be required, but generally, muscle gain is going to be optimally achieved during a phase where weight is increasing over time and fat-loss is likely to be optimised when losing body weight over time.

There are also cases where you may be moving too quickly in the direction that you wanted to, and again, adjustment would generally be advised. In the case of fat-loss, losing weight too quickly can mean that you're not supplying adequate fuel to allow for optimal performance, and gaining weight too quickly can lead to excess body fat gain. Again, other factors, such as visual progress and subjective assessments of sustainability of current calorie level should be taken into account, but generally bodyweight moving faster than recommended tends to lead to diminishing returns over a longer period. There is a really useful decision tree included at the end of this chapter to make this super simple for you.

How Much to Adjust by?

If you've deemed it important to adjust your intake based on all of the above, you'll want to know by how much. There are a multitude of factors at play here, but from experience, a 5-10% adjustment is usually sufficient. E.g., For someone consuming 2500 kcal, this would be an adjustment of 125-250 kcal. This range will depend on various factors, including how far off you are from your goal rate of progress (Is your bodyweight moving in the right direction, but too slowly, or is your bodyweight moving in the wrong direction?), and where your current hunger levels are (If you're already hungry often, decreasing by a large amount is likely to lead to increased hunger levels, and potentially a less sustainable approach).

In terms of macronutrients, this change in calories will generally be achieved through a decrease in carbohydrates, rather than fat or protein. The reason for this is that protein and fat recommendations are generally recommended based on one's body weight, as outlined in previous chapters, whereas carbohydrate intake recommendations are partially based on the fuelling requirements, and therefore have a bit more flexibility when it comes to adjusting them. However, there may be cases where adjusting only carbohydrates leads to increased difficulty in sustainably adhering to the macronutrient targets, in which case, adjusting fat (or in rarer cases, extending that to protein) could be an option. An example of this would be someone who is in a weight-gain phase while being extremely active, who may require a large calorie intake. By increasing their intake by increasing carbohydrates alone, they may be needlessly making it more difficult for themselves, compared to if they'd given themselves a bit more flexibility in food choices by increasing the fat content slightly. On the other end, someone decreasing their food intake might end up decreasing carbohydrates to the point that food volume decreases significantly, meaning they end up being hungrier, in which case, decreasing your fat target could allow for some extra carbohydrates to remain part of the diet whilst still hitting the total calorie target.

Another Option: Adjusting Your Output

Rather than needing to decrease the amount of food you are taking in, another option is to increase the amount of energy you are expending. You may want to do this through introducing some extra running or cardiovascular work into your week, but if your training load is already high, you may be adding to the stress placed on your body, and therefore reducing your recovery capacity. In this case, you can increase activity through tracking your step-count, using a watch or smartphone, for example. Once you've tracked that for a few days, you can increase your step-count target by 1000-2000 per day, which likely lead to an increase in energy output, and therefore assist in fat-loss, perhaps without decreasing energy intake. Alternatively, this could be used in conjunction with altering your calorie intake, reaping the combined benefits.

The Decision Tree

The decision tree below illustrates the concepts above in the context of considering adjusting your intake targets based on your progress. This should be done on a weekly basis, or perhaps a fortnightly basis, using an average of about 4-7 weigh-ins per week (at similar time and situations), in order to even out some of the daily fluctuations that are often seen. It's worth noting that there is an element of both a science and an art to this, so a combination of the objective markers (body weight, for example) and subjective markers (visual progress from mirror or progress photos) will be useful, as will the experience you'll get from going through this process over time, during your journey towards improved body composition and performance.

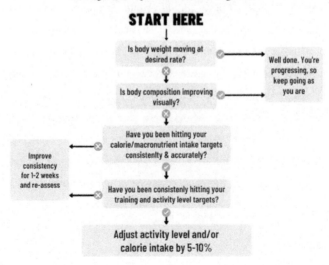

Adjusting Your Food Intake Based on Body Composition Progress

START HERE

Is body weight moving at desired rate? → Well done. You're progressing, so keep going as you are

Is body composition improving visually? → Well done. You're progressing, so keep going as you are

Have you been hitting your calorie/macronutrient intake targets consistenlty & accurately? → Improve consistency for 1-2 weeks and re-assess

Have you been consistenly hitting your training and activity level targets? → Improve consistency for 1-2 weeks and re-assess

Adjust activity level and/or calorie intake by 5-10%

Action Point

Adjusting Your Intake

Each week, or every 2 weeks if preferred, go through the decision tree, and adjust as recommended.

CHAPTER 5:

MICRONUTRIENTS & FIBRE

In previous chapters, you should have calculated your calorie and macronutrient targets, and whilst you will tick quite a few of your nutritional boxes by hitting these targets, the addition of adequate fruit and vegetable intake, as well as a few other alterations, will improve the quality of your overall diet, and look after the smaller, but just as important aspects of your nutrition, which will be discussed in this chapter.

Fruit and Vegetables

The mention of fruit and vegetables probably brings back memories of parents telling you to eat them up if we're going to get dessert. And if you're like many people, that's probably stuck with you, even though you might have let your intake of them fall by the wayside when you began having more control over your own food intake.

Particularly when we know the importance of energy balance and macronutrient intake, it can be very easy to forget about the fundamental importance of fruits and vegetables. But have you ever stopped to ask yourself why fruits and vegetables might actually be important? There are some solid reasons, and knowing these reasons might be what you need to actually start taking your intake of them seriously.

1. They Help with Digestion

Fruits and vegetables are usually high in fibre, and having sufficient fibre intake is important for optimal digestive function. But that isn't limited to your ability to use the toilet. To digest food is to break it down, so that you can get the nutrients out of it, to be used in the body. You can't get the glucose from complex carbohydrates, or the amino acids from protein, without first breaking them down, for example. Soluble fibre (from foods like the flesh of apples and pears, berries, oats, beans, nuts, seeds etc.) form a 'gel' with the food, which may slow down the movement of food through the digestive system, allowing your body to absorb the nutrients in that food. On the other side, insoluble fibre (from foods like fruit skin, leafy vegetables, broccoli, bread, brown rice etc.) provides the food with bulk, accelerating the body's drive to pass the food through, allowing the removal of the food after we've gotten the nutrients from it. For these reasons, in order to make sure the food is travelling through the digestive system at the adequate rate, it's important to consume plenty of both types. Luckily, most fibre-rich foods, even the ones mentioned above, contain some of both forms. Eating a wide range of fruit and vegetables, (whilst adding in other high-fibre foods like whole grains) can go a long way towards optimising your fibre intake. As a side note, fibre intake is also associated with controlling cholesterol, as well as helping reduce the risk of bowel cancer. As a general recommendation, 10g of fibre per 1000 kcal consumed is a good place to start, meaning that someone consuming 2500 kcal daily would aim to eat 25g of fibre per day.

2. They Keep You Full

For many athletes, hunger isn't much of an issue, due to their relatively large calorie intake, but some still struggle with it, particularly when eating less in an effort to lose weight. Given the fact that most fruits and vegetables are relatively low in calories compared to their volume, including more can mean eating more food volume, without adding a lot of calories, and even reducing calories. There was a study done where some of the participants ate an apple 15 minutes before a meal, which resulted in them eating less food (fewer calories) than a group that didn't eat the apple. This basically meant that eating the apple before the meal and then eating the meal, led to less overall intake than eating the meal alone! The study also compared apple juice, which didn't reduce the overall intake, indicating that the fibrous element of the apple probably contributed to the fullness. And you don't even need a study to make this point. If you had a meal of chicken and rice for example, but decided to add a big pile of lettuce and cucumber to the side (basically negligible calories), you probably know without trying it, that it's going to fill you up more.

3. They Provide Micronutrients (Vitamins and Minerals)

It's not quite clear whether or not athletes should be recommended to eat more micronutrients than non-athletes. Some say that the increased demand on the body requires more micronutrition, whilst others say that the usually increased food intake of athletes means that they end up getting more in anyway. Either way, we can say that athletes shouldn't be slacking on their micronutrient intake. There is also some evidence suggesting that athletes are at a greater risk of being deficient in certain specific vitamins and minerals, especially when they restrict their diet in terms of energy (calories), or in terms of specific foods like meat and dairy.

Vitamins are essential nutrients that the body usually cannot produce enough of, and which it needs to get from food. These include the fat-soluble vitamins, A,D,E, and K, the water-soluble B vitamins, and vitamin C. They facilitate a huge number of varying roles within the body, including energy production, cellular repair, skin health maintenance, improving immune system function, among many other things. Minerals are also crucial to maintaining the overall health and functionality of your body. These include things like sodium, potassium, magnesium, chloride, calcium, iron, and zinc, among others. These are also involved in many functions in the body, including fluid balance, the transmission of signals to muscles, muscle contractions, maintenance of structures like bone, and hormonal regulation. It would be much too complicated to start trying to find out how much of each vitamin and mineral you are taking in (although a blood test to find out if you have low levels of specific nutrients might be an option), so instead, you should follow recommendations around your consumption of certain foods, primarily fruits and vegetables. You've likely heard of the 5-a-day recommendation, and it's a good place to start, but getting up towards an 8-10 portion of fruit and vegetables per day mark might be a better place to aim for, given that you are likely to be consuming a lot more food than most people anyway given your energy demands, and because there may be more demand for micronutrients, given the extra stress on your body. Outside of fruit and vegetable intake, consuming red meat 1-2 times per week (for nutrients like iron, for example), consuming oily fish 1-2 times per week or taking a fish oil supplement (for essential omega-3 fatty acids for example), consuming dairy (where possible, for calcium for example), and getting sunlight often (for vitamin D production) can also help ensure adequate micronutrition. A multivitamin can also help, and specific vitamin/mineral supplements can be used to counteract potential deficiencies, but these shouldn't be seen as an alternative to consuming fruits and vegetables.

4. They Help with Hydration

Given that water makes up over 50% of your body, and that water is being removed throughout the day via urination/excretion, breathing, and sweating, it is crucial that we are replacing it, by consuming sufficient water. Doing so allows the body to better regulate its temperature (which is crucial during training), digest food, transport nutrients around the body, lubricate joints, and improve many other biological processes. As an athlete, where you tend to be training often and hard, and therefore tend to sweat more than non-athletes, it can be difficult to meet your hydration requirements through water alone. Many fruits and vegetables can help out here. Some fruits and vegetables are even made up of over 90% water, meaning that whatever volume of that fruit you consume is almost equivalent to consuming that volume of water. e.g. if you eat a piece of watermelon the size of a glass, that is almost the equivalent of drinking a glass of water.

Some fruits/vegetables that are over 90% water are:

- Watermelon
- Cucumber
- Strawberries
- Spinach
- Broccoli
- Melon

Apart from the replacement of fluids, proper hydration also depends on having adequate electrolyte balance. Electrolytes are salts that are often found in foods and drinks, and they include sodium, potassium, calcium, chloride and magnesium, and these are often abundant in many fruits and vegetables. They play a key role in the electrical signalling systems in the body that affect the heart, muscles, and nerves, and they also help regulate fluid balance in the body. Recognising this role in helping you contract muscles during athletic events is often a good motivator for athletes to start getting more fruit and vegetables in.

5. They Keep Your Diet Interesting

At some stage, you've probably been in the habit of eating bland chicken and rice, or plain porridge, or potatoes and meat. It's easy to end up narrowing your range of foods down to a set of 2-3 protein sources and 2-3 carbohydrate sources. If you're someone who loves food, that just gets boring after a while. Who can blame you for feeling the need to eat pizza and take-away food all weekend if you're eating tasteless, boring food all week?

Including fruits and vegetables opens up a huge range of possibilities within your diet. They're extremely versatile, meaning there is a range of different ways that they can be prepared and cooked, so watery, soggy broccoli isn't your only option here. There are also so many different types of fruit and vegetables, that you're sure to find some that you like. You may, however, be asking, "What if I don't like vegetables?". Well, the thing is, you didn't always like things like coffee or alcohol, for example, either, but your taste buds have probably adapted to enjoy these things, or some other food that you didn't used to like. In the same way, your tastebuds can adapt to enjoying vegetables over time, if you eat them enough. However, in order to improve your ability to enjoy them, try preparing them in a few different ways (frying, roasting, raw etc) and try adding spices and sauces to them. A great place to start is to identify those fruits and vegetables that you do like already, even if it's only one of two different options, and include them more often in your meals. From there, you can start to experiment with options that are similar to them, adding them bit by bit, and letting your taste buds adapt. You'll eventually find a variety that you like, and you can then emphasise these within your diet whilst always keeping an eye on bringing more in over time.

Action Point

Fibre, Fruits, and Vegetables

Divide your calorie target (from chapter 1) by 100 to get your fibre target in grams: _____g

How many portions of fruit/vegetables will you aim for per day? _____

CHAPTER 6:

MANAGING APPETITE

Decreasing Hunger

First thing's first: If you are in a phase of fat-loss, where you're likely going to be decreasing your food intake, there are likely going to be times where you're hungry, and it isn't a bad thing. Being hungry doesn't necessarily mean you're losing muscle, or doing yourself any other harm. With that said, if you're *always* hungry, you're likely to make poorer food choices, and ultimately end up abandoning your nutrition plan, so it's something we want to manage effectively.

From an evolutionary perspective, hunger is part of the body's process for motivating us to seek out food, ultimately so that we can survive. In the parts of the world where most people reading this will be, there is an abundance of food, and so, we rarely use hunger as our signal to eat. When, and how much, we eat is usually determined by things like habit, social convention, desire, and convenience. On the other hand, when you are aiming to lose fat, you will usually be eating slightly less than the body optimally would like, so there is a certain amount of restriction involved, which can lead to hunger. With that said, there are a few things we can do to try to limit the amount of hunger we feel, which will likely lead to you being more likely to stick to your nutrition plan over the long term.

1. Eat Enough Food

One possible reason that you're struggling with hunger may be that you're being too extreme in cutting out food, leading to a constant feeling of restriction, and constant hunger between meals. This often comes from an impatience, and wanting to make progress as quickly as possible. A situation like this almost always ends up with a weekend blow-out, undoing a lot of the progress from during the week, leaving you wondering why you haven't been making progress up to this point. When you start eating an amount of food that allows you to make steady, predictable progress, whilst enjoying your food and not starving yourself, then that feeling of needing to eat the house down at the weekend goes away, and you make more progress even with (or likely because of) the less extreme approach.

2. Plan Your Meals

Which of the below options sounds most like you?

1. You go to bed, knowing what you're going to be eating the next day, at what times, and you know it's going to be exactly what you need to hit your body composition and performance goals.

or

2. You'll worry about it tomorrow, and hopefully be able to get your hands on something decent, but aren't really sure what or when.

I'm sure you'll agree that it seems obvious which of those are going to get results with your nutrition approach. But for so many, number 2 is the norm. Then what happens? You wait until you're hungry, then go grab the most convenient thing you can find, which often isn't a great choice. Or, because you feel you can't find anything "healthy", you decide you'll just get something later, or you opt for a protein bar to keep you going. Ultimately, it's a miserable experience, and you get home and justify eating everything in sight, because you've not eaten all day, or you go out to training hungry and under-fuelled, and have a poor session. This brings up a deeper point made famous by a former marine called Jocko Willink, and that is "discipline = freedom". It sounds silly at first, but when put into this context, someone who takes option 1 (the more disciplined approach) actually has more freedom to happily go about their day, knowing their nutrition is sorted, because they've been disciplined in planning ahead. Starting with this might be as simple as making a plan this evening for what you're going to eat tomorrow. It won't be perfect, but it'll put your mind at ease and you'll be more likely to make better choices. You can then adapt and change it as the days go on.

3. Alter Your Food Choices

Why are fruits, vegetables, and protein sources praised as the ultimate health foods? Of course, there are the micronutrients from the fruit and vegetables, and the muscle-building and recovery benefits of the protein. But more than that, in a world where there is an abundance of hyper-palatable (tasty), calorie-dense foods, these foods can offer more filling/satiating alternatives, which can lead to consuming fewer calories, whilst eating a higher volume of food. For you, as an athlete, if trying to drop some weight, these foods should be a big part of your diet. This will help keep you full and satisfied, whilst keeping the diet interesting and allows you to eat a larger volume of food. Even if you're trying to increase your calorie intake, you should still aim for adequate intakes of these foods, for their other benefits as mentioned in previous chapters.

4. Keep Hydrated

There will be more about hydration in later chapters, but amongst the wide range of reasons to keep hydrated is its effect on hunger. Often, the same symptoms can be seen with dehydration as with hunger (e.g. headache, tiredness, irritability). So what you perceive as hunger may simply be thirst! If you mistake this signal, you may end up snacking and adding to your daily food intake, when all you might have needed was a glass of water. Aim to drink enough to have regular clear urinations through the day. 2.5-3.5L is a good place to aim for, biasing some of that to before and after training. All fluids (apart from alcoholic drinks) contribute to hydration levels, including tea and coffee, as well as the water found in foods like fruits and vegetables, for example.

5. Get Enough Sleep

Studies have shown that people who hadn't gotten adequate sleep were more hungry and more likely to choose higher-calorie food options. This obviously isn't ideal for someone trying to reduce their food intake. Even if you are trying to increase food intake in an attempt to gain muscle, please don't take this as a reason to sleep less. Studies have also shown the effects of lack of sleep on muscle gain, and the results were not positive. More on this in future chapters.

Just because you're getting your nutrition on point doesn't mean you should be feeling hungry all the time, and implementing some of these steps may help you reduce the prevalence of hunger, and therefore allow you to enjoy your food, and stay on track with your nutrition.

Getting More Food in

Anyone who struggles to lose weight, and has never been in the position of having to eat more food (in order to gain weight) will likely be envious of the person who is. But if you've ever struggled to eat enough, you'll likely know that it's not as easy as eating everything you want. You obviously want the food you are eating to be of good quality, and you don't want to just over-indulge all the time and gain unnecessary fat. Not to mention, you can sometimes feel that you are force-feeding yourself, eating when you don't feel like eating, all in the name of gaining some muscle and fuelling your performance. However, there are a few things you can do to make it that bit easier to hit your high food intake targets.

1. Track Your Foods

"What gets measured gets managed", and if you're not tracking your food, you're going to struggle to manage and adapt the amount you are eating. Eating 'more' is hard to quantify without tracking how much you are actually eating. Using an app like 'MyFitnessPal' or 'Chronometer', as mentioned previously, you can track your calorie and macronutrient intake, and therefore you can clearly see if you are actually eating as much as you think, and adjust if needed.

2. Schedule Your Meals

Often, athletes who tend to struggle to gain weight, are the same athletes who tend to deprioritise meals when they're busy. Scheduling meals allows you to plan ahead, get organised, and ensure you are eating when you're supposed to. This helps you avoid having to reach for quick, less ideal options on the go, as well as allowing you to plan out meals that allow you to hit your intake targets.

3. Use Liquid Calories

Liquid calories are usually less filling than the equivalent calories/macros from solid food, allowing you to get more in, without feeling as full. Think of apple juice versus an apple. There are roughly the same amount of calories within a medium glass of apple juice as in 2 apples, yet the apples would fill you up a lot more than the juice. You can use this knowledge to get more calories in, by including some drinks/smoothies with your meals, and in between meals.

4. Vary Your Food Choices

Eating similar foods consistently isn't a bad idea in general, as it tends to improve consistently within a diet, but when we include more flavours in our meals, we tend to eat more, which is useful for those with that goal. This is partly why you usually end up eating more food at a barbeque, where there is often a wider range of flavours, textures, and food options, than you would at the dinner table. You can use this tactic to your advantage by including more flavours and textures in your meals, as well as increasing the variety of meals you eat.

5. Include Some Junk Food (within reason)

Eating 3000+ kcal from the likes of chicken, rice, and broccoli every day can become difficult even for the most dedicated clean eater. Food can become boring, and fullness can lead to not eating enough. This is why it can be a good idea to include some foods that you can easily eat and enjoy, that also allow you to hit your calorie/macro intake. Don't take this as a reason to abandon healthy eating habits, but at the same time, don't be afraid to add in some cereal, sweets, chocolate, or pizza every now and then, if your nutrition is solid otherwise, and if doing so allows you to hit your macronutrient and micronutrient targets more easily.

Action Point

Managing Appetite

What tactics will you put in place to manage your appetite, should

you need to?

CHAPTER 7:

HYDRATION

Fluid balance: Fluid out vs. Fluid in

When talking about hydration, it's useful to think in terms of fluid balance, meaning the difference between the fluid that is going out of your body vs. the fluid that you are taking in.

Fluid Out

1. Sweat

Even the fittest of bodies is surprisingly inefficient in terms of energy use, and a huge amount of energy is wasted as heat, especially during intense exercise. It's critical that we dissipate (or get rid of) this excess heat, in order to maintain normal body temperature, or else body temperature would rise extremely quickly, affecting vital biological processes. When we sweat, the sweat evaporates, and carries the heat energy away from the body,

71

into the air (imagine the steam evaporating from a pot of rice, where the heat energy is being taken away from the rice into the air), helping to maintain the body temperature at a safe level. That is all to say that the purpose of sweating is to cool us down. As athletes, we can sweat out litres of water during training sessions and matches, and the amount will depend on various factors, including your physical attributes, activity intensity, length of the activity, and environmental heat and humidity.

2. Urination/Excretion

Urination is one of the body's mechanisms for getting rid of waste products, controlling blood volume and controlling the amount of electrolytes in the body. These are all tightly regulated, and don't need a huge amount of conscious effort on your part, apart from the few recommendations given later around altering fluid consumption. The amount of fluid that you lose through urination (and excretion) is largely dependent on the amount you drink/eat, as well as being affected by other aspects like electrolyte levels and how much you are sweating.

3. Breathing

Fluids are also lost through breathing (the air we breathe out is high in water vapour). Breathing will be affected by training in that we'll be breathing out more air during training as training intensity and length increase.

Fluid In

The fluid we take in can be in the form of water and other beverages, as well as some foods, like fruits and vegetables, which tend to have quite high water content. Consuming sufficient fluids is crucial for athletes, in order to match the fluids being lost through sweat, urination, and breathing, or we risk seeing the negative effects outlined below.

Negative Effects of Dehydration

1. Heart Rate

There was a study done that assessed two groups of athletes in the same running session. One group consumed water during the session and the other didn't. The results showed that heart rate was significantly higher throughout the session in those who didn't consume water, indicating that the same exercise session was more strenuous when under-hydrated. This is backed up by numerous other studies. The proposed reason for this is that as you lose fluid, your volume of blood decreases, meaning the blood is more concentrated and thicker, and therefore the heart has to work harder to pump it around the body, as it aims to circulate nutrients and remove waste products, leading to negative effects on performance as the supply of nutrients to the muscles becomes harder to maintain.

2. Temperature Regulation

As mentioned earlier, sweat helps regulate body temperature by dissipating heat from the body i.e. it cools us down. When you're dehydrated, the body adapts by sweating less, and therefore the body will either increase in temperature to the point of causing harm, or you will be forced to reduce intensity due to the discomfort of overheating. Either case will result in performance being diminished!

3. Electrolyte Levels

Electrolytes are electrically charged particles, which are involved in carrying electrical impulses around the body, and are therefore involved in the nervous system and contracting muscles, both of which are extremely important for athletes. They are also involved in maintaining hydration levels in and out of the body's cells. The electrolytes include sodium, potassium, chloride, bicarbonate, calcium, phosphate, magnesium, and others, all with their own functions. We lose some of these through sweat, and if we don't replace them and they get too low, we can see issues with muscle cramping, fatigue, and ultimately a downturn in athletic performance, or worse than that, health risks.

The Rare Case of "Over-Hydration" (Hyponatremia)

There have been cases, mainly during long-duration endurance events, where people have had serious health issues, and even died, after drinking too much water during the event. Although they were following wise advice in replacing the water they were losing through sweat, they were consuming far too much water, and they weren't also replacing the electrolytes lost through sweat, resulting in the sodium content of the blood becoming diluted, which leads to complications with cell swelling. This isn't a likely concern for GAA athletes, as in general they typically find it difficult to consume a lot of water during training and matches due to the constraints of the sport. However, this example shows that there is a limit to how much you should be drinking, so taking in multiple litres of water in directly before a match or at half-time, for example, isn't going to be a good idea, and sipping on water throughout is a better idea. It is also important to point out that when you are drinking a lot of water, for example during an intense championship match in the summer heat, it's probably a good idea to add some electrolytes to your water, either in the form of a pinch of salt, or an electrolyte supplement, in order to replace the electrolytes lost through sweat.

Practical Implications

All of this might have you feeling unsure as to what you need to do with this information. The good news is that the body is extremely good at regulating hydration levels, as long as a few criteria are being met. If you drink too much, your body will excrete more. If you consume too much salt, your body can usually adjust, and so on. The main thing you have to do is to avoid the extremes of drinking very little, or drinking huge amounts.

With that said, performance usually goes down at about 2% water loss, and thirst usually starts between 1-2%, meaning that if you turn up to a training session or match feeling thirsty, you are already selling yourself short, as it is usually difficult to drink enough during the session or match to match the amount you are losing through sweat and exhalation, resulting in further dehydration and further performance detriment. So one crucial step is to ensure you don't show up to training sessions and matches feeling thirsty.

General Daily intake

The amount you should drink will depend on a lot of factors, but generally about 1L per 25kg bodyweight (E.g., 3L for a 75kg athlete) will be a good starting point, along with seasoning your food (providing salt) and eating plenty of fruits and vegetables, in order to ensure adequate electrolyte intake. Urine colour should also be monitored, ensuring regular, light straw coloured, urinations throughout the day.

During Training/Matches

During training sessions and matches, a good starting point is to simply consume fluids at natural break, aiming for 1-2 mouthfuls every 10-15 minutes, with slightly more during half-time. This drink should generally be made up of water, with some electrolytes, and perhaps some carbohydrates (no more than 7% concentration) which can help with the gut's absorption of the fluid, as well as allowing you to gain the performance benefits associated with carbohydrate supplementation (more on this in later chapters). This tends to be exactly the composition of most sports drinks, and now you know why!

After Training/Matches

After training sessions and matches, it's important to start the rehydration process soon, which should involve sipping on either water and other fluids in the hours after the session, aiming to get back to your previous bodyweight soon afterwards.

Action Point

Hydration

Divide your bodyweight (in kg) by 25 to get your water intake target (in litres) per day: _____L

What other changes will you make in order to affect hydration, based on this chapter?

CHAPTER 8:

SLEEP

There's a spike in car crashes on the last weekend of March every year. Why? Because time "springs forward" by an hour, and we all lose an hour of sleep. That's how important sleep is. In 2014, the U.S. Centre for Disease Control declared insufficient sleep as a public epidemic. So with the general population suffering from not getting enough sleep, you can imagine how athletes, who put their bodies under more stress than most people, can be affected. You may think "It's fine, I can get through without enough sleep" but the problem with lack of sleep isn't just that you feel more tired all day (although you'd think that would be enough to you to get enough sleep), it's that it affects your performance, fat-loss, muscle gain, and general health.

Performance

Studies have been done to investigate the differences in the performance outcomes in people who got different amounts of sleep, and they found that people who got less sleep experienced greater perceived exertion (training/workouts felt harder), lower time to exhaustion (they ran out of steam more quickly), and slower reaction times. As you can imagine, none of this is great for athletes, where these things are crucial. That might be the difference between you outrunning your opponent in the last 10 minutes of the game, or having the concentration levels to kick that important score to win the game.

Fat-loss

Sleep deprivation not only increases hunger levels, but also makes high-calorie, hyper-palatable food, (typically referred to as "junk food") more attractive to us. More specifically, brain scans show that activity in the reward centres increases more in response to junk food when someone is sleep deprived. So whilst sleep doesn't necessarily directly affect fat-loss, it can definitely affect your food choices, which obviously has a major effect on fat-loss.

Muscle Gain

There was a study that compared two groups over a series of weeks: one that slept 5.5 hours per night, and one that slept 8.5

hours per night. Over the course of the study, the first group experienced 55% more fat-gain, and 60% more muscle loss, despite both groups eating the same number of calories. Muscle gain is dependent on putting a stimulus on the muscle, and then allowing it to recover. If you skimp on sleep, you reduce both the stimulus and recovery sides of the equation, and majorly sell yourself short in terms of muscle gain.

Health

Lack of sleep can also have a huge effect on health. In addition to the aspects already mentioned, also affected are things like memory, inflammation, testosterone levels, growth hormone levels, and immune system function. Getting sick keeps you out of training, which means less time practicing your skills, getting fitter and staking a claim for your place on the team.

How Much Sleep Do You Need?

Studies suggest that the required amount of sleep varies a lot between individuals, but 7-9 hours is about right for most people. There is an interesting old-school technique for finding out how much sleep you need: Take a 1-2-week testing period (like a holiday, for example), where you go to sleep at the same time every night, without setting an alarm. You'll probably sleep a lot in the first few nights, as you catch up on the sleep debt you've built up, but as time goes on, you should start to wake up at about the same time each day. The amount of time that you sleep waking up naturally is likely to be the amount of sleep that is optimal for you. This isn't a scientifically validated method, but logically makes sense and could be worth trying.

Tips For Better Sleep

With the negatives outlined in the chapter, hopefully you are convinced that addressing your sleep is an important element of your overall approach, and are ready to take on some tips for improving your sleep. It's not just about the amount of sleep you get. It's also about the quality of that sleep. There are a few proven ways of improving the quality of your sleep.

1. Sleep in a Cave.

'Sleeping in a cave', refers to the idea of making your room as dark as possible, as quiet as possible, and cool (cool enough that you'd need to put a t-shirt on to be comfortable outside of the bed covers).

2. Avoid Screens

Screens like the T.V., laptops and your mobile phone emit a type of light referred to as 'blue light'. The brain recognises this in a similar way to the sun, and since the body's sleep-clock (or more technically, circadian rhythm) is partially controlled by exposure to sunlight, the systems that would otherwise be telling your brain it's time to sleep, won't do so, and you may struggle to fall asleep or your quality of sleep may suffer. Having a cut-off time one hour before bed can help reduce this issue.

3. Have a Bedtime Routine

Why do some people have a pre-match routine? At least in part, it's because they know that that routine puts their body and mind into the right state to undertake the task at hand. So, we know that routines can affect our mental state. The same is true when it comes to sleep. A good sleep routine will put our body and mind into the right state to fall asleep and get into a deep sleep. Again, this will vary for each person, but generally, it should involve things that progressively relax you. Some suggestions would be foam rolling, easy stretching/movement, reading a book, drinking caffeine-free tea, writing, chatting to someone, having a bath etc.

4. Have a Stimulant Cut-Off Time

Caffeine can take about 5 hours for half of it to leave your system, meaning that it could affect your sleep for even longer than that. For that reason, restricting coffee or other caffeine products after mid-day in order to optimise sleep is advised. Nicotine is another stimulant that should be avoided in the evening. Alcohol can also have an adverse effect on sleep. Of course, it can initially make you fall asleep more quickly, but as time goes on, during sleep it tends to act like a stimulant and hamper your ability to get into a deep sleep.

It's been said recently that sleep is the best sports supplement available (and it's free!). Hopefully you can now see why that might be the case.

Action Point

Sleep Checklist

☐ Ensure your sleeping environment is dark, quiet, and cool.

☐ Have a cut-off time in the evenings from screens and electronic devices.

☐ Create a bedtime routine.

☐ Have a stimulant cut-off time.

CHAPTER 9: HOW MANY MEALS PER DAY?

The issue of meal frequency is hotly debated in the nutrition world, often without reference to adequate and appropriate science. On one side, you'll have proponents of eating 6-8 meals per day referring to 'stoking the metabolism', and on the other, you'll have proponents of intermittent fasting, referring to the increased fat utilisation during an increased fasting period when often only eating 2 meals per day within a given window. Both approaches make sense logically on the surface, in different ways, and people have definitely used these techniques to make huge amounts of progress in different fields. But the fact that both of these extremes 'work' should tell you that there is something else underlying what determines your progress. Hopefully having read the earlier chapters of this book, you'll have a good idea of what that might be.

Does it Actually Matter?

Many scientists have studied this area of nutrition and of particular interest here, there have been many studies comparing what happens when two groups of people eat the same number of calories, but one group eats them from fewer meals and one group spreads them out across many meals. The result in the vast majority of these studies is equal outcomes in weight-loss and fat-loss for both groups, when calories are equal. The results of these experiments indicate that what determines outcomes in terms of fat-loss is the calories consumed daily rather than the number of meals one consumes.

With that said, when people are allowed to eat freely (not aiming for a calorie target), studies have shown that people who eat fewer meals per day often tend to see more fat-loss. Think about that for a moment. Does that contradict the previous paragraph? When you consider that when people eat fewer meals, they often tend to eat fewer calories, you'll see that it actually backs up the previous point. When calories are reduced, fat-loss occurs. By removing a meal or two out of your daily intake, most people end up automatically reducing their calorie intake, and losing body fat as a result. It's also important to point out that for other people, reducing the number of meals they're consuming can lead to extra levels of hunger during the period between meals, leading to less adherence to the diet, and ultimately less progress as a result. This leads to the ultimate conclusion that how many meals you eat isn't as important as most people might presume, at least in terms of fat-loss. For these reasons, it's important to assess what meal frequency works for you as an individual from a preference and sustainability point of view.

When it Does Matter

Because of what's outlined above, you'll see many coaches and athletes stop there, presuming that's the end of the story, and that there is no relevance of meal frequency to your athletic goals. But a closer look at nutritional science (and your own practical experience) will tell you that there are a number of elements to consider.

Appetite Management

As I'm sure you can imagine, eating 2500 kcal from 7 small meals is going to feel subjectively different than eating 2500 kcal from 2 large meals. That's not to say one is better than the other. On one hand, you never have to go for any longer than a couple of hours without food, but each individual meal may not be very satisfying/satiating due to the small size. On the other hand, you get to eat 2 large meals, each of which might be very satisfying/satiating, but you end up with prolonged periods of the day where you're not eating, potentially leading to hunger and the propensity to make food poor choices that comes with that. There are pros and cons to both these approaches. However, what's going to suit most people is to eat a number of meals somewhere in between these, where you're able to eat decent sized meals without going for long periods of not eating. Given that there is no real advantage (apart from preference perhaps) to having a very small or very large number of meals outside of the normal range, opting for somewhere between 3-5 meals/snacks tends to be a good starting point for most people in terms of keeping hunger minimised and allowing for enjoyable meals. This tends to make sense for most people's daily lives also, having breakfast, lunch, and dinner, and perhaps a snack or 2.

Schedule

When it comes to any intervention in your life, it has to work within the framework of your overall existing lifestyle. For example, if you're a busy professional working 60 hours a week, your ability to choose when you eat or train is going to be limited in comparison to a student who only has classes for 16 hours of the week. For that reason alone, a blanket recommendation of a number of meals per day won't be broadly applicable to everyone. One person may only have 2-3 opportunities during the day to eat, whereas another might have complete control of their time and be able to eat 5-6 times if they wanted to. Finding a meal timing strategy that fits into your daily schedule will make a big difference to how easy or difficult making the changes feels, and therefore how sustainable your approach will be. Getting this right will usually involve planning and trial and error, in order to get that number right for you.

Muscle Protein Synthesis (MPS)

Muscle Protein Synthesis is the creation (synthesis) of muscle tissue, that occurs when we eat a sufficiently large, high-quality protein source, and/or when we engage in resistance training (lifting weights, for example). The body is constantly in a state of both breakdown and synthesis of all of its tissues, and muscle is no exception. For this reason, optimising the synthesis (building) side of that equation is crucially important for your recovery and muscle/strength gain goals. Logically, it would make sense to aim to 'spike' this MPS response as many times as possible per day. However, studies have shown that aiming to do so any more than about 5 times per day doesn't bring any extra benefit. The same research also showed that 'spiking' the MPS response 3 times per day brought close to the same daily total benefit per day as 5 times per day, when the same total protein intake was consumed for that day. This leads us to the conclusion that eating 3-5 protein sources per day is optimal for increasing muscle protein synthesis, and therefore helping optimise your recovery and muscle gain. This obviously isn't possible if only consuming 1-2 meals per day, and also indicates that eating more than 5 times per day isn't required, so eating 3-5 protein-containing meals per day is recommended.

Eating Around Training and Matches

As you'll see in upcoming chapters, getting your nutrition right around training and matches can have a big effect on your performance, as well as your recovery and adaptation. For this reason, both the pre-training and post-training meals should be seen as a key part of any nutritional approach. If you're only eating 1-2 meals per day, this may make it more difficult to optimise these meals, since it will require that you eat a lot of food within each of them. Adjusting your eating schedule to allow you to optimise those meals will likely require eating more than 1-2 meals per day, again, making the 3-5 meal per day target as a good one.

Action Point

Choosing Your Ideal Meal Frequency

Think about how many meals per day would likely be ideal for you, given your current lifestyle and schedule. With the knowledge that 3-5 meals per day is recommended as optimal, decide on a how many meals per day you are going to eat going forward. As you implement this, adjust as needed based on what works best for you, allowing you to manage your hunger levels, hit your calorie and macronutrient targets, consume adequate amounts of high-quality food, and optimise your meal timing approach around training and matches, all whilst fitting into your daily schedule.

CHAPTER 10:

EATING ON TRAINING

VS. NON-TRAINING

DAYS

It intuitively makes sense to eat more food on days where you're completing energy-intensive training sessions vs. days where you're not training or have sessions that require less energy provision. The idea is that you want to provide the body with more fuel for the sessions where it's needed. But you also know, based on what you've read so far, that adding in extra food on those days will increase your weekly energy intake, and perhaps interfere with body composition goals you may have, particularly if fat-loss is a goal. Even if fat-loss isn't a goal, however, you'll still recognise an issue here in questioning how much extra you should be eating on training days, and if you should be adjusting your intake elsewhere.

At the crux of it, as with most of the guidance in this book, you want to be able to walk that line between doing what is right for performance and improving or maintaining a certain body composition. In this case, you'll want to be able to provide the body with the fuel needed for what you're asking of it, closer to when it's needed, whilst also not increasing total energy intake for the week. This is sometimes referred to as 'calorie-cycling'.

Defining Your Days

In order to maintain your energy intake targets for the week, it is important to compensate for any increase in calories on training days with a decreased amount on non-training days. In this case, you can consider 'training days' as those days where you're training with the team or where you're doing tough running/cardio-based sessions alone. You can then count non-training days as those days where you're not training at all, or those days where you're doing gym sessions or other similar sessions that, while tough, aren't going to demand the same energy requirements as those of running sessions. This might change for athletes for whom strength is strength or other gym-based activities are their key sessions, where these might then be counting as training days. In exceptional circumstances, you could have 3 different daily intakes, but this would be excessive in most cases, without much benefit, so 'training days' and 'non-training days' is sufficient for GAA players to reap the benefits of this approach.

Should You Use This Approach?

So, should you implement this approach? The first thing to consider here is the previously mentioned concept of 'consistency over perfection'. In this case, even if a calorie-cycling approach is deemed beneficial technically, if doing so leads to confusion and inconsistency through the week for you, a simpler approach of keeping your calorie intake consistent each day is likely to lead to better outcomes. If in doubt, start with a period of a few weeks where you're keeping calories consistent every day before moving to this approach where it differs on training vs. non-training days.

Another factor that matters when it comes to deciding if this approach is suitable for you is your current body composition goal. Someone who is in a fat-loss phase, where the energy intake they are currently taking in is leading to weight-loss, is likely to benefit most from calorie-cycling, since it will allow them to be close to a maintenance level of calories on training days (providing adequate calorie intake for the work required), whilst being in a larger calorie deficit on days where they aren't training, allowing them to see fat-loss over time as a result. Someone who is currently eating at maintenance level (where body weight is staying stable across weeks on average), is also likely to benefit, since they will be able to stay at the same weight, whilst having extra calories for fuel on training days. Someone who is currently eating at a level that has them purposely gaining weight (i.e. they're eating in a calorie surplus) is not likely to benefit much from this approach, since they're already eating excess calories that can be used as fuel, both on training and non-training days.

How Much Extra Should You Eat?

Again, there are numerous factors at play here, such as how low your calorie intake currently is and if you're currently experiencing hunger on a regular basis (bringing calories even lower on numerous days per week is likely to increase hunger levels). A 10% increase on training days tends to be a solid approach. This figure is by no means fixed in stone, but is based on experience with athletes as well as what logically and logistically makes sense - An extremely small difference of say 2% would be unlikely to make any difference in terms of the effects you're hoping for, and a much larger amount like 25%, for example, would likely lead to excessively low intakes on non-training days. Increasing your calorie intake on training days by 10% means that if your current daily intake (calculated in chapter 1) was 2500 kcal, that would increase to 2750 kcal (2500 + (10% of 2500)) on training days.

You could simply leave it at that, increasing your intake on training days, and leaving your intake at the regular level on non-training days, but that will lead to an overall increase in your daily average calorie intake across the week. If, however, you wanted to maintain your average daily calorie target for the week, then you need to adjust your non-training day intake downwards in order to even out the average. If you are training 3 days per week, and therefore eating that new 2750 kcal target 3 days per week, you've just added in an extra 750 kcal (250 x 3) to your weekly calorie intake. In order to ensure your average daily intake for the week remains the same as it was before, you then need to take those extra calories out of the other 4 days of the week. That can be done by simply dividing that extra 750 kcal by 4, since there are 4 non-training days: (750 / 4 =187.5 … Call it 190 kcal for ease of maths and practicality), leaving your non-training day intake at about 2310 kcal (2500 - 190) and training day intake at 2750 kcal. (Note: Don't worry if that was confusing. There's a super simple calculation at the end of the chapter).

Of course, your calorie intake will likely be different than the 2500 kcal in the example above, and you may want to experiment with increasing or decreasing that 10% figure, but hopefully the maths example shows you how you can match it to your needs and goals.

Adjusting Your Macronutrients

In general, any changes in calorie intake on training vs. non-training days should be reflected in carbohydrate intake as opposed to protein or fat (this is why sometimes this approach is called 'carb-cycling' rather than 'calorie-cycling'). The reason for this is that the body's protein requirements generally stay the same on a day-to-day basis, as does fat, and recommendations for both of these are generally based on your body weight, whereas the body's carbohydrate requirements generally change based on your energy output demands. It also logically makes sense since carbohydrates are the main energy source used in high-intensity training. There may be exceptions, where fat or protein will be also changed slightly, but they are few and far between. An example of this would be where calorie intake has become so high that it becomes too difficult to get all the extra calories from carbohydrates alone, and increasing fat as well might be a good option.

As a final note, many athletes have achieved their body composition and performance goals whilst keeping their calorie intake consistent through the week, without the need to change for training vs. non-training days, so consider the calorie-cycling approach as an optional extra, if and when it is implementable on a consistent basis for you.

Calculating Your Training vs. Non-Training Day Intake

Here are the steps for you to take to calculate your training day vs. non-training day targets:

1. Enter your daily calorie target (from chapter 1): _____kcal

2. Calculate 10% of answer 1: _____ kcal

3. Add answer 2 to answer 1 to get your training day calorie target: _____ kcal

4. Multiply answer 2 by the number of 'training days' you have per week: _____ kcal

5. Divide answer 4 by the number of 'non-training days' you have per week _____ kcal

6. Minus answer 5 from answer 1 to get your non-training day intake: _____ kcal

Your calorie intake targets:

Training days (answer from number 3): _____

Non-Training days (answer from number 6): _____

To find your new macronutrient targets for training vs. non-training days, add/subtract from your carb targets by dividing the calorie difference by 4 (since there are 4 calories per gram of carbohydrates). E.g. 100 kcal divided by 4 = 25g of carbohydrates.

CHAPTER 11:

CARBOHYDRATE

LOADING

It sometimes seems that carb-loading is touted as the be-all and end-all when it comes to performance nutrition, in spite of the poor implementation often seen. On the other hand, most players have never really tried it, beyond maybe having some pasta the night before a match. And although it clearly isn't the only thing we should be worried about, it is worth delving into what it is, and where it should or shouldn't fall into your nutrition plan.

Carbohydrates for Sport

When you're making those blistering runs back and forth up the pitch, or doing tackling grids in training, the body needs to create energy quickly to keep up with those demands. It also needs to be able to do that for a sustained period of time. The optimal fuel source for this job is glycogen. When you eat carbohydrates, they are broken down into glucose, which is circulated around the body via the blood, and ultimately stored as glycogen in the muscles. This glycogen is then available for use during intense activities, like those we see in training and matches. The more glycogen we have available in the muscles when it comes to match-day, the more fuel there is available, and hopefully, the better our performance will be, or at least a poor performance won't be because of lack of fuel!

What is Carb-Loading?

Carb-loading (or carbo-loading or carbohydrate-loading) is a term used to describe a strategy used to increase the amount of glycogen (stored carbohydrates) within the muscles for a sporting event, by increasing carbohydrate intake in the days leading up to that event. The original method proposed involved a few days of very low-carbohydrate intake (with a lot of training to deplete stores), followed by a few days of extremely high carbohydrate intake (and no training). As you can imagine, however, this was logistically quite difficult. On match-week, all you want to do is focus on getting to match-day, but here, you're looking at 7 days of changing your diet, with each of those 7 days being different from your usual intake, and with the presupposition that you have complete control over your training load. Sure, if you thought there was no other option and that it was going to help a lot, you'd probably do it, but fortunately, researchers compared an approach of simply increasing carbohydrate intake in the 1-3 days leading up to the event, and found that this was probably just as effective as the approach of going from very low-carb to very high-carb days.

Who Does it Work For?

The research, such as that just mentioned, was done mostly on endurance athletes, who obviously have different demands than GAA athletes. The former involves staying at a relatively steady pace for a long time, whereas the latter involves mostly short, intermittent bursts followed by short recovery periods. With that said, both significantly deplete glycogen stores, particularly at higher intensities. For that reason, maximising glycogen stores is likely to be beneficial for GAA sports. At a very basic level, given that glycogen is the predominant fuel source in high-intensity activities, performance will be improved by having sufficient stores to pull from. With that said, it's probably not as necessary for a GAA athlete as it would be for a long-distance runner, since it's unlikely that a GAA athlete is going to completely deplete his/her carbohydrate stores during a match, but having high glycogen availability can improve athletic performance, and it's better to have the stores there for when they're needed, also because it tends to be a much better fuel source than fats or muscle protein.

How to Do it

In terms of practical application, simply increasing carbohydrate intake in the 1-2 days leading up to match-day will likely be sufficient. For some, this may simply be a case of adding in a large portion of carbohydrates to each meal, or adding in a couple of extra high-carb meals/snacks. For those who want to bring in a bit more accuracy, and have been tracking their food intake as outlined in previous chapters, consuming 5-8 grams of carbohydrate per kg body weight (400-640g for an 80kg player) is recommended. For those who are new to tracking their food, this can be tracked through the MyFitnessPal phone app or other apps. This intake might seem very high for many people, and if that is the case, you can always start at a lower intake and you're still likely to get some benefits if it's above your usual intake. You can then increase over time as you get used to it. There are also cases where someone with a fat-loss goal may not want to increase their carbohydrate intake, since this may increase their calorie intake significantly for the week, potentially decreasing their fat-loss for that week. That will be an individual decision based on the balance of their fat-loss and performance goals. In this case, a more practical method might be to increase your carbohydrate intake slightly the day before a match, opting for closer to 4g per kg bodyweight rather than 5-8g.

On a practical level, the usual sources of carbohydrates (potatoes, rice, pasta, oats etc.) will be good options. However, I would highly recommend opting for mostly lower-fibre options if you're eating very high amounts of carbohydrates, as well as bringing in some higher glycaemic options (breakfast cereals, sports drinks, sugary sweets, juices) for reasons outlined in the next section, but also because players often find it difficult to get enough carbohydrates in when they are eating very filling sources.

Avoiding Common Mistakes and Problems

There are a few common problems that tend to come up with carb-loading approaches, and the first thing to mention is that you should practice it a few times beforehand, in the weeks/months leading up to match-day, so that there are no surprises when it comes to doing it for match-day.

It's Not an Excuse to Eat Whatever You Want

Carb-loading shouldn't be used as an excuse to eat whatever you want. It shouldn't be used as an excuse to overeat on pizza and pastries the night before a match or event. Instead, it should be viewed as a strategic approach to improving performance. Yes, you will be eating more food, but the likelihood is that you will have to make a conscious effort to eat enough and to eat the right types of foods. When carb-loading, you should increase your carbohydrate intake, but keep your fat and protein intake constant, or as close to constant as possible. You want extra carbohydrate stores in the muscle, and adding in extra fat intake isn't necessarily going to help with that, but will provide additional (potentially excessive) calories, on top of the already high levels. In order to manage this, we want to be looking at carbohydrate-dense sources, like rice, pasta, potatoes, cereals, breads, as opposed to things like pizza, pastries, foods with creamy sauces, and deep-fried foods, which do tend to contain carbohydrates, but also contain a lot of fat. Even having some of the foods usually thought of as poor food choices, like breakfast cereals, sugary sweets, and fruit juices can be used here as easy-to-consume sources of almost completely carbohydrates.

Digestive Issues

Any major change to the diet is likely to cause digestive issues, as the gut tends to adapt to what you feed it consistently, at least to a certain extent. Even if you were to majorly increase fibre intake (fibre is generally seen as a good addition to the diet), the gut would struggle to deal with it, and you may experience digestive issues. In that case, it would be important to gradually increase fibre intake and allow the gut to adjust. The same can be true for carbohydrate intake. It is important to 'train the gut' over time to be able to handle the high-carbohydrate intake that you're asking it to process, so start low, practice outside of preparation for important matches, and improve your approach over time based on what you feel works best. This can be done by eating a relatively high amount of carbohydrates in general, but also in practicing carbohydrate-loading for training sessions, or less-important matches in the weeks leading up to the game.

Gut issues can also occur as a result of eating too much fat, fibre, or protein during the carb-loading process. This is easily done when increasing carbohydrates, as you may feel the need to increase all of your food sources. However, it is important to keep fat, fibre, and protein intake under control, and increase carbohydrates alone. It can also be a good idea to opt for fewer of the whole-grain type carbohydrate sources during the carbohydrate-loading period, since these will inevitably have a higher fibre content.

Another, often overlooked, issue is stress, which can result in gut discomfort. This is often unavoidable to some degree, which is why players often prefer to have a lighter meal before a match, increasing the importance of having done most of the fuelling up in the previous days.

Action Point

Calculating Your Carb-Loading Targets

Calculating Your Carb-loading Targets:

1. Multiply body weight in kg by 5-8g: _____ - _____ g
2. Compare this to your usual carbohydrate intake and choose an amount within the above range that seems practical to you (or slightly lower if the above seems extreme compared to your usual intake).
3. Increase or decrease this over time based on your experience and practice.

CHAPTER 12:

THE PRE-MATCH MEAL

"It was 5pm on the day of an under-age GAA match. 17-year-old me looked through the kitchen cupboards and fridge, trying to put together a pre-match meal. I guess I must have read somewhere, earlier that week, that carbohydrates were the body's preferred energy source, and decided that the more of them I could eat, the more energy I would have for that night's match. This led to the 'obvious' meal choice of two packets of microwaveable basmati rice, with nothing else, except a touch of sweet chilli sauce, for taste. After chomping through the bulk of the rice, I slumped in the chair, wondering how this feeling of bloated, drowsiness would eventually lead to me performing at the top of my game in 2–3 hours, but still, I trusted that this information I'd read was factual and that this feeling would ease off by the time I got to the game. It didn't. With the rice still lodged in my stomach, and still feeling no surge of energy, I sat in the changing rooms before the match, wondering what I'd done wrong. Needless to say, the game passed me by, and

any energy I had was used trying to stop myself from throwing up."
Everyone has their own pre-match or pre-event meal disaster story,
and most people have tried many different combinations of meal
timing and meal content, but it's time to start dialling in a better
approach.

It's Not Just About the Pre-match Meal

Looking at the stages of preparation from a nutritional
point of view, the general diet in the weeks and months leading up
to the game shouldn't be overlooked, so it is worth mentioning that
even the most optimal pre-game meal is not going to make as big a
difference as addressing the diet in general. Doing so will allow you
to have optimised your body composition and created good habits.
Making sure the general diet is on point is crucial, and you'll have
done a good job of that having followed the advice in previous
chapters. It's also important to remember that the "fuelling" period
for a match goes beyond that meal you have a few hours before the
match. It's important to also start thinking about the days that lead
up to the match, and considering implementing the carb-loading
approach from the previous chapter will guide you on how to
achieve this.

Game Day

Obviously your match-day food will be affected by a lot of different things, including the time of the match, whether you're eating at home or with a team, and even how nervous you are feeling on the day. During a time where there are many variables at play, it is improtant to control as much as you can, meaning that you should prepare ahead of time, having bought any food that you need in the days beforehand, having planned out what your meals and snacks are going to be, getting out of bed at the right time, and so on. The aim with your game day eating is to top up glycogen stores, achieve adequate hydration, and generally feel energetic going into the match. Outside of the pre-match meal, your game day meals should generally contain some carbohydrates and protein, with moderate-low amounts of fat and fibre, and no foods that you know you don't digest well, in order to avoid any digestive troubles, and snacks should be mostly carb-based, again, topping up the glycogen stores. Hydration should also be a priority, sipping on water throughout the day, without going majorly over your usual intake.

The Pre-Match Meal

If you've done everything mentioned above, you're almost good-to-go in terms of getting your nutrition right for game-day. The last step is that period of a few hours before the game, right up to the starting whistle. There are two periods worth thinking about when it comes to pre-match nutrition. The first will be the final set meal before going into the match, and the second will be the period of about an hour before the match.

1. 1-4 Hours Pre-Match

In the 1–4 hours before the match, the aim is to make sure you are topping off glycogen levels in the body and increasing blood glucose levels appropriately. That means consuming some form of carbohydrate. However, eating a carbohydrate-only meal would not be optimal. Having a protein source, such as chicken, for example, and a small amount of fibre in the form of vegetables or fruit, will slow down the rate of breakdown of the carbohydrate, keeping your blood sugar levels more stable. This protein feeding also has the advantage of supplying amino acids, which will then be present during the training session or match, decreasing the amount of protein (muscle tissue) being broken down to be used as fuel. This effect may be small in the overall context, but another advantage is that this may also help the recovery process post-competition. In this meal, you may also want to avoid slow-to-break-down foods such as fats and fibre, since you'll want to avoid the feeling of a full stomach during competition. The size of the meal will vary greatly for individuals based on how soon before the match the meal is being eaten (obviously smaller the closer to match time), the size of the individual, whether or not they had meals earlier in the day, personal preference, potentially how nervous they are (nerves making it difficult for some people to eat, or even digest their food) and a few other factors.

Generally, a meal in the 1–4 hours pre-match should consist of some form of slower-digesting carbohydrates, such as rice, potato, sweet potato, oats etc, with some form of lean protein such as chicken, turkey, lean beef, dairy, whilst avoiding foods high in fat and fibre (That may mean not having a big pile of vegetables in this meal.)

A few examples of pre-match meals:

- Seasoned chicken with rice and spinach
- Oats and whey protein with a banana
- Baked potato and turkey mince with a handful of berries
- Sweet potato with lean beef with rocket leaves
- Pasta with chicken and a moderate amount of tomato sauce

  (All of these meals should be seasoned with some salt, as there will be a loss of salts during the match, and these will help with fluid balance and hydration.)

Timing-wise, recommendations will be quite different based on your individual situation, but generally, the final set meal should be between 2-4 hours pre-match, allowing adequate time for the food to be digested, but not so far away that you are hungry before or during the match. If you have your pre-match meal 3-4 hours pre-match, it could be worth snacking on some carb-based snacks in the hour or two leading up to the match. Good examples would be rice cakes, toast, fruit (dried or fresh), and oat bars (be careful of fat content).

2. 0-60 Minutes Pre-Match

In the 0–60 minutes before the match, which may include the period during or after the warm-up phase, you may want to take advantage of the chance to get some extra glucose into the bloodstream, potentially topping up some glycogen stores and lessening the onset of fatigue. This can be done through some form of concentrated carbohydrates, such as jelly sweets, or dextrose, glucose or maltodextrin powder mixed with water, or perhaps an isotonic sports drink or gel, if the budget allows for this. Sipping on a drink pre-match can actually help with hydration as well, particularly by adding a pinch of salt or electrolytes to the mix, since this helps replace some of the electrolytes that will be lost through sweat and helps regulate fluid balance/hydration. (These electrolytes/salts are already contained within isotonic sports drinks for this reason.) You should be mindful of the potential for this drink to affect performance through creating a feeling of nausea, as well as creating the need to use the toilet during competition, so some experimentation is required. The next chapter on intra-performance nutrition will talk more specifically about this type of drink.

Another potential supplement to consider pre-match is caffeine. This will be covered in the supplements section, but essentially, it can be beneficial to consume caffeine pre-match or pre-training, for an extra cognitive and physiological boost. It is important to consider timing and dosage. Caffeine generally peaks in the bloodstream about 45 minutes after consumption, so altering intake based on that can be beneficial. The recommended dosage is 100-400mg (more on this in the supplement chapter). As well as that, it is important to consider how caffeine affects sleep. Caffeine can remain circulating in the bloodstream for over 5 hours, so if consuming caffeine for an evening match or training session, it's important to factor this in, and alter the timing and/or dosage as needed, knowing that poor sleep can have a major negative effect on recovery, health, hunger levels, and general well-being.

Action Point

Your Pre-Match Meal Checklist

☐ Plenty of carbohydrate and water in the days leading up to the game and on game-day.

☐ Pre-match meal containing carbohydrates and protein.

☐ Limit hard-to-digest foods (high fat and fibre foods) in the pre-match meal.

☐ Eat at a time that allows you to not feel hungry or full during the match.

☐ Consider a pre-match drink containing some concentrated carbohydrates and some salt or electrolytes.

☐ Consider supplementing with caffeine 45-60 mins pre-match for a cognitive and physiological boost.

CHAPTER 13:

INTRA-PERFORMANCE

NUTRITION

In this context, the prefix 'Intra-' refers to that time within the period of the match (or perhaps training session) itself, and more specifically, that time from the start of the warm-up until the moment the training session or match finishes. There are a few things that you should consider within that window in order to optimise your performance, as well as your adaptation/recovery from that session.

Fuelling

The first thing that we can influence in the intra-performance period is the aspect of fuelling. If you've already adequately 'fuelled up' through carbohydrate loading and an appropriate pre-match/training meal, then you can think of this intra-performance fuelling as the cherry on top of the cake. It is worth noting, as has been mentioned throughout previous chapters, the idea of consistency being more important than perfection, meaning in this case that if starting to think about fuelling during training and matches seems overwhelming, or you haven't yet been consistently hitting your other nutritional targets consistently for a decent period of time, then it would likely be better to focus on those more foundational aspects first, leaving the intra-performance aspects for down the line. With that said, exercise bouts of over 60 minutes have been shown to deplete glycogen stores somewhat, potentially leading to decreases in performance levels. These decreases in glycogen stores have also been associated with increases in muscle protein breakdown. By providing replacement for some of these glycogen stores through consuming carbohydrates during the activity, you will potentially be able to avert these issues, thereby helping performance and reducing muscle breakdown. Research suggests that for those engaging in endurance events lasting over 70 minutes, consuming 30-60 grams of carbohydrates every 15 minutes in order to maintain glycogen levels is close to optimal. However, given the intermittent nature of GAA sports, as well as the lower amount of time generally involved, we can assume that GAA athletes require less than distance runners, and opting for 30-60 grams per full intense training session or match is probably closer to the requirements of a GAA player. This may increase or decrease for longer training sessions or matches that go to extra time, or one-day tournaments for example. This can be consumed through a combination of sports drinks, carbohydrates powders, energy gels, sugary sweets, and other options (check out the supplements chapter for more on these). It is worth noting that these options vary in digestibility, which will also depend on the individual's response. It's also worth noting that there is research suggesting that for most people, the limit of how much carbohydrate the gut can consume is about 1g/minute on average, which coincides with the above recommendations. However, this is worth experimenting with for yourself, as it will be an individual matter. It is also possible to 'train your gut' to be able to process more carbohydrates over time, so starting off with low amounts and increasing them over time is a recommended approach.

Hydration

The second aspect to consider is hydration, and this is connected to the fuelling aspect, since, as you'll have noticed, many of the carbohydrate sources are delivered via liquid. When it comes to hydration, as with fuelling, you should aim to be coming into the training session or match already adequately hydrated, seeing the intra-performance aspect as a means to maintaining that, rather than it helping you simply get back to baseline. Fluids tend to be lost during training sessions and matches via sweat and breathing (and perhaps even the half-time toilet break). When internal fluid levels decrease, problems with temperature regulation and electrolyte levels tend to occur (more on this in the hydration chapter). Again, by providing adequate levels of fluids and electrolytes during performance bouts, you can help to ameliorate those potential issues. The amounts of fluids and electrolytes required will depend on the intensity of the session, the temperature of the weather, and the individual's sweat rate, but a solid recommendation is around 250ml every 15 minutes. Some research suggests that the gut can't process much more than about 1 litre per hour, so limiting your intake to this level is likely a good idea.

Protein

We've talked about carbohydrate intake, as well as fluid/electrolyte intake, but a third element to consider is protein intake. Generally, adequate protein intakes spaced throughout the day will be sufficient to cover your recovery and muscle adaptation needs. However, protein intake during intense training has been shown to improve glycogen replenishment, decrease muscle damage, and decrease muscle protein breakdown for fuel, especially when combined with carbohydrates. Carbohydrate ingestion during training may be enough to do this alone, but due to potential time constraints and potential absorption/digestive issues, the addition of protein can be useful. For the purposes of the usual length of a training session or match, it is likely not necessary however, particularly if you have consumed a protein-rich meal in the hours leading up to the training session or match, and if you will consume a protein source shortly afterwards. If deemed necessary to consume protein intra-training (for example, if you weren't able to consume a protein source within the hours beforehand, or if the session is longer than usual in cases such as a one-day tournament) 20-30g of protein in the form of whey or other protein powder is recommended. An EAA (essential amino acids) supplement can be used in place of a protein powder during activity if digestion of protein powder is problematic for you, but again, this is likely not needed with adequate protein beforehand, or carbohydrate intake during the performance bout.

The Ultimate Home-Made Intra-Performance Drink

Given all of the above, you can consider making our own intra-performance drink, consisting of a carbohydrate powder, electrolytes (in the form of supplement or perhaps even just a pinch of salt), whey protein or an EAA powder (if deemed a requirement), and water. Other supplements, such as caffeine and creatine, can be added in here if you're taking them regularly anyway (more on this in the supplement section). This is something you can start sipping on from the start of the warm-up right through to the end of the training session or match where possible, or if more practical, you can drink half of it during the warm-up, and half at half-time, or better yet, space it out in 15-minute intervals. The addition of some sugary sweets or energy gels could be experimented with also, if the additional carbohydrates are needed. The use of these elements in particular requires you to pay particular attention to digestion, assessing how increases or decreases in various elements suggested affects how you feel. Starting off with low amounts and building up over time is advised, and practicing this approach in training sessions before trying them out in matches is crucial in order to avoid any unwanted stomach upsets or otherwise when it matters most!

Train Low?

There is some recent research showing the potential to increase fitness adaptations by training with low glycogen stores and low carbohydrate intake during training. This may seem contradictory to the recommendations above, but it isn't necessarily. It's important to recognise the difference between adaptation and performance within a specific session. In the case of 'training low', the likelihood is that performance within that session might actually be worse, but the fitness adaptations may actually be better (consider the idea of wearing a weight-vest during a running session. You wouldn't be able to run as fast, but you may actually get a stronger fitness adaptation off the back of that session. The same could be said for training in a glycogen-depleted state in some cases). Whilst this is quite recent and limited research, and is something that is of such minute detail compared to other aspects we've gone through throughout this book, it's still worth considering for future reference. Given this, I don't recommend that you consistently and consciously aim to train (or certainly play matches) with low glycogen stores or carbohydrate provisions. Instead, a better approach might be to only use the intra-training approach discussed in this chapter (particularly the carbohydrate intake) for matches, or training sessions where optimal performance is required. This might have to be balanced by the desire to impress management in every training session in order to give yourself the best chance at getting your spot in the team, so this will be very much an individual decision, based on these factors. Again, if this seems overly complicated to you, file it in the section of 'not required right now'.

Intra-Performance Checklist

- ☐ Consider 30-60g of easily digestible, fast absorbing carbohydrate, spread out across the match or training session, in the form of carbohydrate powders, gels, sports drinks, sweets, etc.

- ☐ 250ml of water every 15 minutes on average. Consider adding electrolytes in the form of a supplement or a pinch of salt.

- ☐ Consider 20-30g of protein in the form of whey, or an essential amino acids supplement if adequate protein intake wasn't possible in the pre-training meal.

CHAPTER 14:

RECOVERY NUTRITION

The definition of recovery is, "returning to a normal state of health, mind or strength." In the context of sport and athletic training, this means that you want to be able to train, and after a rest period of usually 24-48 hours, be at the point where you're able to repeat the previous training session with equal or greater intensity. That is to say, we want to create a stressor on the body, and allow the body to recover and adapt to that stressor. Over time, this allows your body to handle more work, as the muscles and other systems become stronger and more enduring. This effect can be seen in the following graph, where the line moves down with each training session, signalling fatigue, but moves upwards between sessions, signalling recovery and adaptation.

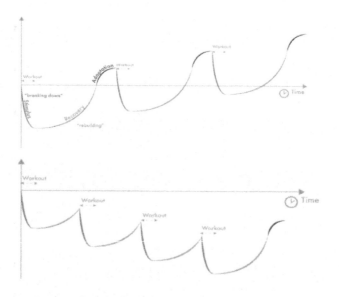

The issue is that when you don't allow for adequate recovery and adaptation, whether that is through inadequate rest, inadequate time between sessions, added life stressors, or poor nutrition, you go into that next training session under-recovered. If this is repeated chronically, over time, it can lead to diminished performance, fatigue, and often, injury. Hopefully that starts to put into context the post-training meal, and its importance at a time where the body is most fatigued, but also shows that it isn't the only important aspect, since the recovery and adaptation period is much longer than the hour or two after a training session. If you've ever done a hard training session, you'll already know that the recovery isn't done only in the hours after training, and your sore (still recovering) legs the morning after will let you know that.

Recovering

As mentioned, the aim of nutrition between sessions is to help you get back to a state where you could repeat the session with similar or greater intensity. This is done by allowing for recovery and adaptation, as well as refuelling. There are a lot of things that we can do to affect this, including sleep/rest, interventions like ice baths, and even different types of recovery sessions, which can be discussed at a later point, but here I want to specifically talk about nutrition.

Rebuilding

The first nutritional aspect to consider when It comes to recovery is protein. As you'll know from previous chapters, protein is broken down in the body into amino acids, and these amino acids can be seen as the building blocks of muscle tissue (among other bodily tissues). Given the stress placed on the body and muscles during training, the demand for these amino acids is high after training sessions, particularly if it's been a while since your last protein feeding. This is, in part, due to the fact that the muscle tissue will have been partially 'broken down' during the training session, which we will want to counteract, by providing protein and therefore signalling a Muscle Protein Synthesis (MPS) response, where the body will signal the creation of new muscle. The body requires around 25g of protein from a good quality source in order for this to happen, and this can be optimally signalled about 3-5 times per day. This is one reason why the thought that "the post-training meal or snack is all that matters for recovery" is false. That is only one opportunity to signal this MPS response, and it is important to continue to signal this in the meals that follow. In terms of timing, a common thought is that you need to get a protein shake in as soon as your foot touches the changing room floor after the session. This is potentially a good thought taken too far. Whilst, as we mentioned, we want to take the opportunity to get some protein in soon after training, waiting 30-60 minutes after finishing the session will likely be no problem, which may be a relief if you've felt the discomfort of trying to eat or drink something immediately after a really tough training session. It may, in fact, by preferable, since the blood flow in the digestive system will be greater 30-60 minutes after the training session finishes, which can help with the digestion of any nutrients consumed at that point. And of course, this post-training protein feeding doesn't have to come from a protein shake. Whey is a great source of protein, being quickly digested, quickly absorbed, and convenient, but it is only one option, where your usual sources of protein (chicken, meat, eggs, dairy products etc.) are also sufficient.

Refuelling

If you are going to be fully ready to complete the next session to the best of your ability, it is important that you have adequate fuel in the muscles. For the high-intensity training sessions and matches that are common in GAA, the main energy source used will be carbohydrates, or more specifically, the stored form of carbohydrate, known as glycogen. Given that after a training session or match, you'll have likely just used a lot of the previously stored glycogen, it is important to refuel in time for the next session, and that means eating sufficient carbohydrates between sessions. Carbohydrates include the faster-absorbing sources like sports drinks, sugary sweets and some fruits, as well as the slower-absorbing ones that you might have as part of a meal, like potatoes, rice, oats, and pasta, and actually, getting some of both in after training session or matches can usually be helpful in relacing glycogen stored quickly. The exception might be for someone who is aiming to lose weight, where avoiding the faster-absorbing (and therefore less filling) sources might allow you to bias your intake towards the slower-digesting sources, and therefore remain fuller and more satiated with your food. The amount that you eat between this training session and the next will be determined by a lot of factors, including your body weight, your general activity levels, and your body composition goals. For the most part, this will be covered by following the calorie and macronutrient targets you calculated based on the first few chapters of this book.

However, what we do know is that for optimal performance in the next training session, refuelling does need to happen at some stage. It is a good recommendation to start that refuelling process soon after the training session, especially if you are training or competing again within the next 24 hours, in order to avoid struggling to get enough carbohydrates in in the meals leading up to that session. In terms of timing, it probably isn't as important as the timing of your protein, but practically, it's probably easiest to have some carbohydrates with your protein feeding. Carbohydrates consumed soon after training sessions are also more quickly stored as glycogen in the muscle, since there is an increase in insulin sensitivity after intense activity, which is another reason that consuming carbohydrates soon after a session could be useful.

Rehydrating

Water will become depleted during a training session, and should be considered in the post-training period. Being adequately hydrated aids with digestion, blood flow, and mineral balance, among other things. Electrolytes also fall into this category. Since you lose a lot of water and electrolytes during training sessions through breathing and sweating, it is important to try to maintain hydration during the training session, but also to continue to rehydrate afterwards. This can be through fluids like water (potentially with electrolytes), sports drinks, smoothies, and milk products (milk and chocolate milk have both been shown to be very effective for rehydration after exercise). One metric for assessing hydration is to measure how your body weight differs after the session from before, as a result of fluid losses. Aiming to get back close to that weight in the hours following the session through sipping on water and/or the other fluids mentioned above is recommended.

The Recovery "Window"

As a final point, the immediate post-training "window" isn't all you have to worry about with your nutrition, and in fact, isn't a very useful way to think about it. Knowing this is useful in two ways:

1. It means that you have to focus on your overall nutrition, not just one meal after your training session. 2. It means that if you happen to be in a situation where you can't get a decent meal straight after training, all is not lost, since this is not the only meal that affects your recovery and adaptation to training.

Action Point

Recovery Checklist

- ☐ Adequate training load management (not training too much or too little).

- ☐ Adequate sleep and rest.

- ☐ Sufficient protein in general on a daily basis, and 25g+ of protein in the form of a meal or snack within about an hour after training.

- ☐ Sufficient carbohydrate intake in general on a daily basis and carbohydrates in the post-training meals/snacks, especially if training again within 24 hours.

- ☐ Sufficient water intake in general on a daily basis, and increased water intake post-training, with the aim of returning to around the pre-training weight within the hours afterwards, also considering electrolyte supplementation.

- ☐ Considering ice baths and other recovery techniques when appropriate (such as in times where getting recovered quickly is the main aim. E.g. 2 matches in 3 days).

CHAPTER 15:

MEAL PLANNING

A Word on Meal Plans

The concept of meal plans is a contentious one. On one hand, a lot of people come to a nutritionist expecting to receive a nutrition plan that they can just follow meal by meal for the foreseeable future. On the other hand, hopefully you've learnt by now that this is not necessarily going to be the best approach for most people, given the issues with sustainability - Can you imagine eating the same foods every day for the rest of your life? And if not, is a strict meal plan really useful long-term?

With that said, there can be some usefulness in meal plans, in that they give you a structured approach and starting point to what a day of eating could look like in order to hit your specific goals. However, the trade-off is often that you don't go through the process of learning the principles of nutrition, leading to a lack of adaptability, flexibility, and ultimately losing out on the potential to manage your nutrition by yourself.

Rather than seeing meal plans as a strict prescription to follow, a better approach would be to they see them as rough examples of what your diet might look like. Your meals should be made up of foods you enjoy, foods that are accessible to you, and should have an element of adaptability. The tracking process (as outlined in the starting chapters) tends to be a much more flexible and adaptable and sustainable way of approaching nutrition, it spite of it's own downsides, including the extra time and care it takes to do it. After a period of doing this, most people find themselves able to get to a point where they no longer need to track unless they're going into a specific phase of changing their nutrition.

With all that in mind, you'll find some example meal plans in this chapter. Again, these are examples to give you ideas around what your day of eating might look like, but there are no specific foods that need to be included in your meals, nor foods that aren't on this that you should avoid. Spend some time creating your own example meal plan based on your own calorie and macronutrient requirements. Even then, be completely open to this changing on a daily basis, using the food tracking process to include foods where needed based on what's going on that day etc. Also, if using the meal plans provided as examples, feel free to look at those below and above your own calorie targets to get some other ideas for meals you might include, simply adjusting ingredients up or down as needed. Again, I can't emphasise enough, following these meal plans strictly is not recommended. They are simply ideas, and using the food tracking process in order to hit your specific calorie and macronutrient goals is recommended.

How to Plan Your Own Meals

Before looking at the example meal plans laid out, let's look more generally about planning out your meals. Given the GAA player's requirements for protein, fat, and carbohydrates, as well as fibre and micronutrients, you should be aiming to include some element of each of these in each of your meals. A very simple way of approaching that is to pick 1 or 2 sources of each per meal. You'll find examples of each category in the following list, so that you can start piecing meals together based on that. You'll also see that reflected in the example meals plans outlined after that. The amount of each of the foods will depend on your exact calorie and macronutrient requirements, so weighing and tracking your food, at least for a period of time, in order to get an idea of how much you should be eating for your goals, is recommended.

PROTEIN	FAT
Chicken fillets	Olive oil
Chicken (Whole)	Coconut oil
Steak	Various nuts
Minced beef	Seeds
Salmon	Nut butters
Tuna	Butter
Turkey steak	Coconut milk
Turkey mince	Fat on meat
Ham	Eggs (yolks)
Eggs	Avocado
Egg whites	Olives
Tofu	Dark Chocolate
Greek yoghurt	Cheese
Cottage cheese	Chia seeds
Milk	

CARBOHYDRATES	FRUIT & VEGETABLES (fibre/micronutrients)
Basmati/Brown rice	Peppers
Noodles	Onions
Potatoes	Mushrooms
Sweet potatoes	Broccoli
Pasta	Carrots
Oats	Peas
Rice cakes	Asparagus
Oat bars	Beetroot
Granola	Lettuce
Cereal	Spinach
Dried fruit	Oranges
Fruit	Apples
Rice Cakes	Pears
Quinoa	Bananas
Some vegetables	

Example Meal Plans

Below, find outlined some examples of what your daily meals might look like. There are options for various rough calorie intakes. Exact amounts of each food with their calorie and macro amounts have intentionally not been included in most cases, because the aim is to have enough flexibility to allow you to take aspects of each and adapt them to your needs. You'll be able to use those below as rough guides, and through tracking your daily intake and adapting, you'll be able to get closer to your own specific daily targets. Remember, these are examples, and there's no need to think you have to follow them strictly. It's about finding a way of eating that works for your preferences while allowing you to hit your daily calorie, macronutrient, and micronutrient needs, and if the examples below help you do that, use them as needed, and if not, don't.

1750 kcal

Breakfast: 3 poached eggs, spinach, tomatoes, 1 piece of toast
Lunch: Salad with lettuce, sweetcorn, grated carrots, chicken, light salad dressing
Dinner: Seasoned turkey mince with peppers, onions, and rice
Snack: Low-calorie jelly pot

2000 kcal

Breakfast: Porridge with banana and protein powder

Lunch: Bread roll with tuna, sweetcorn, and light mayo

Snack: An orange and grapes

Dinner: Chicken fillet with potatoes and broccoli

2250 kcal

Breakfast: Overnight oats with milk, protein powder, frozen berries, almond butter

Lunch: Baked potato with baked beans and low-fat cheese

Snack: Plain Greek yoghurt

Dinner: Chicken stir-fry with baby corn, mangetout, and rice noodles

2500 kcal

Breakfast: 4-egg omelette with ham, peas, mushrooms, hot sauce, and 2 pieces of toast

Lunch: Wholemeal wrap with chicken, chilli sauce, cheese, lettuce, and an apple

Dinner: Chilli con carne and rice

Snack: 2 rice cakes

2750 kcal

Breakfast: Yoghurt with banana, almonds, granola, and honey

Lunch: Quinoa salad with chicken, peas, baby tomatoes, cashews, raisins

Dinner: Salmon, sweet potatoes, broccoli, and avocado

Meal 4: Chicken Sandwich with lettuce

3000 kcal

Breakfast: Porridge with mixed nuts/seeds, blueberries, banana, protein powder, dark chocolate

Lunch: Pasta Bolognese

Dinner: Homemade chicken curry with rice

Snack: Bowl of cereal with milk

3250 kcal

Breakfast: Smoothie with oats, nuts, frozen berries, banana, protein powder

Lunch: Salmon, peas, sweetcorn, and rice

Snack: Banana and peanut butter on rice cakes

Dinner: Homemade burgers with homemade chips

Snack: Yoghurt with nuts and fruit

3500 kcal

Breakfast: 5 scrambled eggs with 3 pieces of toast, and avocado

Meal 2: Chicken stir-fry with noodles

Meal 3: Fajitas with onions peppers and rice

Meal 4: Protein oat pancakes with dark chocolate and honey

Meal Planning

With the help of the examples given in this chapter, or even disregarding them completely if it's easier, create your own 'ideal day of eating', containing foods that you enjoy, a meal frequency that suits your schedule, and in amounts that allow you to hit your target calorie and macronutrient intake. This exercise will get you used to the tracking process, but will also give you a great idea of what a day of eating should look like suited to your goals. Feel free to create numerous 'ideal days' with differing foods and meals.

CHAPTER 16:

SUPPLEMENTS

There's a reason that supplementation is one of the last chapters of this book. It's because generally it's the first thing a lot of GAA players will go to when thinking of improving their nutritional approach, when in fact, it probably should be one of the last things, given how much relative impact the other aspects talked about in this book will have. With that said, appropriate supplements can have their place. Once you've gotten the bulk of your nutritional approach in order, it can be worth looking at supplementing, to address deficiencies in your diet or to provide ergogenic (performance-enhancing) aids. In this chapter, you'll find a series of supplements that may be useful to you, depending on your situation. As an important note, it is recommended to only use supplements that are batch-tested and certified as free from illegal performance enhancing drugs, so be sure to do your research when it comes to the quality of your supplement provider. Looking for certification marks like those from 'Informed Sport' will help ensure you're covered here.

Please note that this list is not exhaustive, so there may be supplements outside of the list that infer benefits. You also shouldn't feel the need to use every supplement on the list. In fact, adding one at a time will allow you to assess any benefits and correctly attribute them to the supplement. Finally, as with any advice mentioned in this book, speak with your physician before undertaking any nutritional intervention.

Protein Powder

Protein, whether from food or supplements, contains the amino acids needed for recovery and growth of muscle tissue, as well as other tissues in the body, making protein essential for the growth and repair of those tissues. Hitting a sufficiently high protein intake through food alone can be difficult. In this case, a protein powder, such as whey protein, becomes a high-quality, convenient, versatile source of this protein. Although protein powder is usually put in the supplement category, it can be classified as a food, albeit it's gone through various processes and had ingredients added to it. The most popular form of protein powder, whey protein, is actually a by-product of the cheese-making process. It can be added to meals (e.g. porridge oats or yoghurt) or mixed with a liquid (e.g. water or milk) and drunk as a stand-alone shake in order to increase protein intake. Various non-dairy protein powders are also available, and can be used for similar purposes. The serving size is generally around 25g, but this can be increased or decreased to suit your needs. It is often used as a post-training recovery drink, due to its convenience, which is a worthy use of it, but it can be consumed at any time of day.

Carbohydrate Supplements

Carbohydrate supplements also fall into a category somewhere between food and supplement. The main source of concentrated carbohydrates throughout history was honey, and this concentrated source of energy (in the form of carbohydrates) was said to have been used by warriors before going into battle as a n energy aid. Scientists have since done many studies on the effects of carbohydrates on exercise performance, and carbohydrate intake before and during intense training and competition has been shown to be beneficial to performance, through providing an ample energy supply when it's needed most. This is partly why sports drinks have become so popular, and these can be viewed as a carbohydrate supplement. However, there are also less expensive methods of garnering the benefits of carbohydrates in a supplemental form. Glucose, dextrose, maltodextrin, vitargo, and highly branched cyclic dextrin are popular forms of supplemental carbohydrates that can be consumed around training and matches in order to provide that extra supply of energy substrate. These examples usually come in the form of powders or energy gels, for use in various situations, and each have their own advantages and disadvantages. Those who are aiming to lose weight, or even for some people who are trying to maintain weight, might be best served by leaving out or limiting these extra carbohydrate supplements before and during exercise, since the calories therein obviously contribute to one's daily caloric intake, potentially leading to that person having to cut down their food intake elsewhere. However, even swirling a sugary drink in the mouth and spitting it out has been shown to provide some performance benefits. Carbohydrate supplementation is not for everyone, as some people experience excessive blood sugar fluctuations during exercise after excessive carbohydrate consumption. This may also be related to the amounts, and so trial and error will allow individuals to assess this for themselves. Digestive issues can also occur with large intakes of these supplements, although the gut can be 'trained' to handle more over time, so timing and amounts are something to experiment with, if you decide to use carbohydrate supplements. In terms of recommendations, you can start consuming your carbohydrate powder (mixed with water or diluted juice) or energy gel 30 minutes before the workout/session/match, and continue to consume it right through the warm-up, and throughout the activity. Around 30-60g of carbohydrate per hour of activity in total is recommended for sports like GAA, coming from a sports drink, a mixed drink of water with a carbohydrate powder (with flavour from another source such as diluted juice if needed), an energy gel, or other source, such as jelly sweets. There is more information on this in the intra-training chapter.

Creatine

Creatine is a collection of a specific set of amino acids, found naturally in foods like fish and meat, and is also naturally created within the body. It is involved in energy production in activities lasting a short amount of time, where a quick turnover of energy is needed. This includes activities like sprinting, jumping, and lifting weights. It is the most researched sports supplement, and no consistent negative side effects have been shown. Supplementing with creatine monohydrate provides the body with greater stores of creatine than you could reasonably get from food, leading to greater performance in those short, intense activities. This can lead to improvements in power output, strength, speed, and possibly even endurance activities over time. Most GAA Athletes will benefit from supplementing with creatine for the performance benefits, and it would be of particular benefit to those who are trying to gain muscle and strength. The recommended daily dose of creatine is 3-5g per day of the creatine monohydrate form. The creatine stores in the body will become saturated over a period of weeks/months, as opposed to having an immediate effect, so you can take it at any time of day. However, having it at a time of day that you'll remember to take it, such as with breakfast, or in your post-workout shake, can improve your likelihood of taking it regularly, and therefore reaping the benefits.

Caffeine

We all know the wakening effect of a cup of coffee on a tired weekday morning, but the benefits of caffeine consumption can also extend to athletic performance, with increased cognition and muscular performance being seen when taken before exercise.

Its effects on wakefulness are caused by caffeine interfering with adenosine (a molecule that signals sleepiness in the brain), and the more performance-enhancing effects are, at least in part, caused by increases in hormones like dopamine and adrenaline. Caffeine can be used by those who want a bit of a boost before training or matches. It's particularly useful for those who don't usually drink a lot of coffee or other caffeinated products, as it is more effective in people who don't usually use it. However, regular users can get similar effects by taking an increased dose (within reason). General supplementation recommendations for exercise performance are 100-400mg, depending on your tolerance, general caffeine use, and subjective feeling when using it. It's usually best to start off low and increase the dosage if needed, so that you know what to expect (jitters and increased anxiety can be side effects of excessive caffeine intake, for example). Supplementation can be in the form of a cup of coffee, or other supplements like gum, energy drinks, and caffeine pills. Another issue worth considering is caffeine's effect on sleep. It takes about 5 hours for half of the caffeine consumed to leave your body, so it is important to monitor how your sleep is affected, particularly for evening training sessions and matches, adjusting the timing and dosage of your intake as needed. This will vary based on the person, but in general, having a cut-off time for caffeine intake somewhere in the late morning/early afternoon is a good place to start. With evening training sessions and matches, weighing up the performance benefits vs sleep detriments will be a personal decision, but prioritising the sleep aspect, outside of perhaps those most important matches, is likely to lead to better outcomes over time.

Fish Oil

Omega-3 fatty acids are essential in the human body, meaning that they cannot be created within the human body and need to be consumed through food or supplementation. They are found, most notably, in oily fish, but given the lack of oily fish that is eaten today, people tend to under-consume these essential fatty acids compared to what is optimal, and doing so can increase your risk of cardiovascular disease, diabetes, and several forms of cancer. On a lower level, getting sufficient intake of these nutrients can help with recovery and possibly even muscle growth. Supplementing with fish oils in the form of liquids or capsules can be a convenient and effective method for increasing Omega-3 intake. Anyone who is seeking optimal health should aim to consume at least 2-3 servings of oily fish per week, but if this isn't possible or practical, then supplementing daily with fish oils can be a good second option. The recommended daily dosage of fish oils is 1-2g of combined DHA/EPA per day. When selecting a fish oil supplement, it's important to note that this 1-2g recommendation is the combined DHA and EPA amount (usually found on the back of the label), and not the total fish oil amount (usually found on the front of the label). These can be consumed at any time of day but are generally best consumed with food to aid with their digestion. Choosing a liquid version over a capsule version is usually less expensive, albeit that there is a trade-off of having to taste the liquid.

Vitamin D

Vitamin D is known as the sunlight vitamin, due to the fact that our body creates vitamin D when our skin senses sunlight. It is involved in the absorption of calcium and therefore has an effect on bone health, but it has also been shown to significantly affect other aspects of health such as inflammation, the immune system, and even mood. Unfortunately for most of us, it's not practical to get a lot of sunlight, especially in the winter. Supplementation is recommended for anyone living in a part of the world where it isn't often sunny, and/or for those who don't spend much time in the sun. The recommended daily dosage for vitamin D is 1000-4000IU, which can be taken at any time of day, but should be taken with a source of fat, since it is a fat-soluble vitamin. For this reason, taking it with a meal, which will also help you to remember to take it each day, can be a good idea. There is a lot of research showing benefits across various health markers with supplementation of vitamin D, and research continues to show more benefits as time goes on. It is also relatively inexpensive and readily available. For these reasons, it is a supplement very worthy of your consideration.

Magnesium & Zinc

These 2 supplements grouped together here, simply because they are most commonly found together in ZMA supplements, which also contains vitamin B6 (surprisingly though, since it doesn't seem to have any effect). Magnesium and Zinc can be taken as separate supplements, which is generally a better approach for sourcing quality versions in the quantities that you want. Athletes, in particular, are often deficient in magnesium and zinc, and bringing levels back up has a combination of effects including enhanced insulin sensitivity, increased testosterone levels, improved mood, better exercise performance, better sleep, and many other benefits. ZMA supplements are an easy way of getting both Zinc and Magnesium in sufficient doses all in one supplement, but these can be supplemented separately. Athletes tend to be lower in magnesium and zinc, as intense training and sweating can deplete levels in the body. It is recommended for those who are training at a high level, and/or have some other reason to consider themselves at risk of deficiency. Most ZMA supplements contain the recommended supplemental amounts in each serving, which is about 10-50mg for Zinc, and about 200-400 mg for Magnesium (Magnesium glycinate is a form of magnesium with high bioavailability so is recommended). Zinc supplementation at the onset of a cold has also been shown to decrease the duration of symptoms, and magnesium supplementation before sleep has been shown to improve sleep quality.

Vitamin C

Vitamin C is involved in the immune system, as well as in regeneration of connective tissue, and it is also an antioxidant. Supplementation has been shown to decrease the likelihood of getting a cold, for example, as well as the duration of an already present cold. It is generally quite easy to get the recommended amount of vitamin C through the diet, by consuming plenty of fruits and vegetables like oranges, peppers, and greens. For this reason, most people probably don't need to regularly supplement with vitamin C, but it might be worth supplementing with up to 2000mg (spread throughout the day) if you feel a cold coming on, or if you already have one, in an attempt to decrease the length and severity of it. It can also be worth supplementing at times where you would be at greater risk of getting a cold, like during winter, and/or during a tough training cycle.

Multivitamin

Multivitamins contain many of the recommended daily intakes of various vitamins and minerals. With a healthy, varied diet, we can get most of these without the need to supplement. For athletes with particularly high intakes of foods, this ability to hit the recommended intakes can be increased. However, there is also an argument that athletes need more, due to the demand they are placing on their body. We see this with the depletion of magnesium/zinc stores, for example. A multivitamin is by no means essential, but can be a relatively inexpensive means of covering off any potential deficiencies within the diet. However, taking a multivitamin should never be used as a reason not to maintain a diet filled with a wide variety of healthful foods. For those who are in a weight-loss phase, and are therefore likely eating less food, it could also be worth supplementing, particularly if the training load remains high. Another case for supplementation would be for those people who have identified various potential deficiencies in vitamins and minerals that can be rectified by a multivitamin, without the need to buy the various vitamin and mineral supplements separately. There is a wide range of options when it comes to buying multivitamins, but opting for trusted brands and choosing an option the suits your budget, towards the higher end if possible, is recommended.

Beta Alanine

Beta Alanine increases the body's ability to buffer acid build-up in the muscles, particularly in activities lasting 60-240 seconds. For GAA athletes, this can mean delaying the time it takes for the feeling commonly referred to as "Lactic Acid" build-up to occur in the muscles, meaning better performance in training sessions that involve that type of training. This can also potentially help us get out more reps in the gym, leading to greater strength and muscle gains. Beta-Alanine is potentially useful for those who have already optimised their overall diet, are training extremely hard, and have the budget to experiment with an additional supplement. The benefits of Beta-Alanine supplementation occur only after a period of consistent use over a period of weeks, so it's not necessary to take it directly before and workout or training session. Supplementation with beta alanine can lead to a tingling feeling in the skin, which is thought to be harmless, but can be avoided by spreading out the dosage throughout the day, which may also be a more optimal intake in terms of the benefits. The recommended dosage is 2-5g per day.

Citrulline Malate

Citrulline Malate supplementation increases L-arginine levels in the blood, which increase Nitric Oxide Production, which has the effect of increasing vasodilation (the opening of blood vessels), and therefore increasing blood flow. This potentially improves the body's ability to get oxygen, glucose, and other key nutrients to the working muscles whilst also allowing for improved ability to remove 'waste products' from the muscles. It has been shown to be beneficial in terms of reducing fatigue, possibly due to its ability to increase the body's ability to replenish energy substrates (mainly glucose and phosphocreatine). All that is a long way of saying that it increases blood flow, helping the flow of nutrients and energy to the muscles. This is a supplement worth considering for those who have already got the rest of their diet on point, and are looking for something that might bring a small percentage of benefit, if the budget allows for it. It is only likely to show benefit in those who are training hard, and often reaching a point of muscular fatigue. It is also worth noting that the research is mixed, with some research showing lesser effects than others, so it may be worth experimenting with for yourself. The recommended dose is 6-8g (6000-8000mg) around an hour before training sessions and/or matches.

Beetroot Juice

Beetroot juice had a spell of popularity a few years ago, and with decent reason. 500mg of nitrates (from about 500ml of beetroot juice or 1-2 concentrated shots), has been shown to increase exercise performance in both running and cycling time trials, as well as increasing time to exhaustion. This may have some carry over into performance in GAA, with both fatigue and time to exhaustion being important. This effect is most likely due to the increase in Nitric Oxide production in the body, leading to increased blood flow and therefore increased ability to provide nutrients and energy to the working muscles. High-nitrate food like beetroot can be a beneficial addition to your overall diet, so if you enjoy the taste, add them in. Supplementing with them prior to training/matches could have a slight performance benefit in terms of reducing fatigue, so for those who already have the rest of their diet nailed down, and have the budget for it, it could be worth experimenting with. The recommended dose of about 500mg of nitrates, 2-3 hours prior to exercise, can be provided by 500ml of beetroot juice, 500g of whole cooked beetroot, or 1-2 shots of concentrated beetroot juice.

Collagen Hydrolysate/Gelatin

Recent research suggests that consuming gelatin (which is coincidentally the main ingredient used in making jelly), also known as collagen hydrolysate, can help with recovery of joint injuries. Given the high amount of joint injuries seen in GAA, this can be a useful supplement to have in mind to use when needed. Gelatin/Collagen Hydrolysate provides the amino acids necessary for the synthesis of new joint tissue. Given the shortage of blood flow through joint tissue in general, it can be useful to supplement with this shortly before rehab/training sessions where the target joint is going to be used, in order to give the amino acids the best chance of being transported to the recovering area. Although this is a relatively new field of research, those who have joint injuries or general issues with their joints should consider supplementing. Note also, that whilst this product will technically provide protein, it shouldn't be seen as a replacement for protein in the diet, since the amino acid profile is not similar to that protein which contributes significantly to muscle gain/muscle recovery. A 10-15g dose around an hour before an exercise session involving the injured joint has been shown to be effective. Some vitamin C is required along with the gelatin/collagen hydrolysate for joint tissue synthesis, so it is recommended to consume either some fruit juice or a multivitamin/vitamin C supplement along with it.

Action Point

Supplementation

Identify what supplements will you consider using, if any, having read the information in this chapter, given your specific goals and needs.

CHAPTER 17:

BRINGING IT ALL TOGETHER:
THE ONE-PAGE NUTRITION PLAN

1. Based on your goals, what are your daily calorie and macronutrient intake targets? What foods will make up your general meals?

Calories: General Meals:
Protein:
Fat:
Carbohydrate:

2. What are your targets for the below food quality and lifestyle factors?

Fruit/veg portions per day: Hours of sleep per night:
Fibre per day: Daily step count:
Litres of water per day:

3. If and when you decide to have different intakes on training vs. non-training days, what are your calorie and macronutrient intake targets?

Training days   **Non-Training Days**
Calories: Calories:
Protein: Protein:
Fat: Fat:
Carbohydrate: Carbohydrate:

4. If and when you decide to use a carb-loading approach, what will be your calorie and macronutrient intake targets? What changes will you make to your pre-performance meal and intra-performance nutrition, if any?

Carb-Loading Targets
Calories: Pre-performance Meal:
Protein:
Fat: Intra-performance Nutrition:
Carbohydrate:

5. If you decide to use any supplements, which ones?

CONCLUDING REMARKS: IT'S OVER TO YOU

What you've read in this book will remain 'words on the page', unless you go out into the real world and implement it. Information is great, but it would be unwise to expect results from consuming information alone. However, I am 100% confident that consistent implementation of the information you've read here will result in significant progress over time, and with the confidence gained from that, you will implement more diligently and consistently, creating a positive feedback loop that will bring more and more progress. That success in body composition and performance may even carry over into other areas of your life, since progress in one area tends to lead to the self-belief that you can progress in other areas.

That's the real aim from all of this.

Good luck on your journey,

Conor

A Major Favour – And Something Extra for You

If you got anything from this book, I'd massively appreciate that you do one of 2 things:

1. Rate and/or review the book on Amazon. This massively helps more people see the book and get the useful information that you have. Just search 'Fuelling the Gaelic Athlete' on Amazon and you'll find it. Send me a screenshot on any platform once you've done it.

2. Share a photo or screenshot of the book to any social media platform. This could be a photo of the front cover beside your morning coffee, or a snippet from the book, or whatever you feel like sharing. Be sure to tag me @knowyourselfperformance so that I can see it.

If you do either of these two options, either send me a screenshot of the review, or tag me in your social media post, and I'll send you on something special to say thanks. Trust me, it'll be worth the 2 minutes that it'll take you.

Most of all, thank you for your purchase of the book and thank you for reading it.

Where to go From Here

If you have any questions or comments on the information within this book, I'd love to hear from you. Feel free to send me an email at conor@knowyourselfperformance.com, or message me on any of the usual social media platforms (search: Know Yourself Performance).

If you want to find out more about my content, products or services, or want to work with me directly, visit knowyourselfperformance.com.

Bibliography

This book is written predominantly for practical implementation for players, rather than use as a scientific textbook. Whilst the information within has been based on the scientific literature, I've refrained from going into the deep physiology, for example, which would likely lead to overcomplication for those it has been directed at. In the same vein, I've refrained from adding citations throughout the book. However, I'm aware that there will be some readers who are more scientifically-minded, and may want to follow up with some deeper reading into the research. For this reason, I've included a bibliography containing many of the main resources that have helped to inform the contents of this book. This list is by no means exhaustive, but will provide hours of educational content for the keen nutrition enthusiast. In addition to these, if there is any piece of information in the book for which you'd like a reference, reach out to me via email here: conor@knowyourselfperformance.com.

Advanced Sports Nutrition – Dan Bernardot

The Complete Guide to Sports Nutrition – Anita Bean

The Muscle and Strength Pyramids - Andrea Valdez, Andy Morgan, and Eric Helms

Essentials of Strength Training and Conditioning – National Strength and Conditioning Association

NSCAs Guide to Sport and Exercise Nutrition – National Strength and Conditioning Association

Sports Nutrition in Practice – BTN Academy

Journal of the International Society of Sports Nutrition and their position stands – International society of Sports Nutrition

Advanced Nutrition for Mixed Sports – Lyle MacDonald

A Guide to Flexible Dieting – Lyle MacDonald

The Rapid Fat-loss Handbook – Lyle MacDonald

The Ultimate Diet 2.0 – Lyle MacDonald

Optimal Nutrition for Injury Recovery – Lyle MacDonald

Gut – Giulia Enders

Bigger, Leaner, Stronger - Mike Matthews

Fat Loss Forever – Layne Norton

Renaissance Diet – Dr. Mike Israetel et.al

Alan Aragon's Research Review – Alan Aragon

Countless research papers found through Google Scholar and PubMed searches

Most importantly, 1000s of hours of hands-on experience and gaining objective and subjective feedback from the 1000+ athletes that I've worked with throughout the years.

Printed in Great Britain
by Amazon

22987722R00086